W. Brett A. Todorov M. Pfisterer H.-R. Zerkowski   (Eds.)

Surgical Remodeling in Heart Failure –
Alternative to Transplantation

W. Brett A. Todorov M. Pfisterer
H.-R. Zerkowski (Eds.)

Surgical Remodeling in Heart Failure –

Alternative to Transplantation

■ Basel Heart Workshop Series

With 48 Figures and 27 Tables

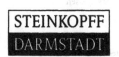

STEINKOPFF
DARMSTADT

Dr. W. Brett   Dr. A. Todorov
Prof. Dr. M. Pfisterer   Prof. Dr. Hans-Reinhard Zerkowski
Universitätsklinik für Herz- und Thoraxchirurgie
Kantonsspital Basel
Spitalstraße 21, CH-4031 Basel

ISBN 3-7985-1223-X Steinkopff Verlag, Darmstadt

Die Deutsche Bibliothek – CIP-Einheitsaufnahme
A catelogue record for this publication is available from Die Deutsche Bibliothek

Steinkopff Verlag is a company in the BertelsmannSpringer publishing group
© Steinkopff Verlag, Darmstadt 2000

Medical Editor: Sabine Ibkendanz – English Editor: Mary Gossen
Production: Klemens Schwind
Cover Design: Erich Kirchner, Heidelberg
Typesetting: K + V Fotosatz GmbH, Beerfelden

SPIN 10749915   85/7231-5 4 3 2 1 0 – Printed on acid-free paper

Foreword

The number of patients with endstage heart failure is increasing worldwide and optimal treatment of such patients will be a major challenge in cardiovascular medicine during the first decade of the new millennium. Heart transplantation in patients with heart failure refractory to medical management has evolved from an experimental approach to the gold standard with excellent long-term survival, allograft function and quality of life when compared to the deleterious natural history of the disease. However, the more widespread use of heart transplantation remains limited by the shortage of donor organs. In addition, the development of chronic graft vasculopathy and malignancies remains an important long-term threat for heart transplant recipients. The development and application of alternative surgical techniques for the improvement of ventricular function in patients with severe heart failure is therefore mandatory.

This workshop held in Basel in August 1999 provided a comprehensive overview on today's available surgical techniques for the improvement of symptoms and prognoses of endstage heart failure. In the first part, new insights into the neurohumoral, molecular and subcellular mechanisms for the development of the heart failure syndrome are presented by G. Hasenfuss followed by extensive reviews on options for medical treatment of endstage heart failure by P. Poole-Wilson and on heart transplantation as a therapeutic gold standard by W. Harringer. The second part gives an overview on cardiomyoplasty techniques by S. Salmons and the Paris experience in this field by J. Chachques. The third part deals with geometrical, hemodynamic and metabolic considerations in reverse remodeling of the enlarged left ventricle by Ch. J. F. Holubarsch and their application and effects on symptoms and prognosis with mitral valve repair presented by S. F. Bolling and left ventricular reduction surgery presented by R. Batista. The fourth part with a review on the clinical application of artificial hearts by R. Körfer and insights in future developments on biomechanical hearts by H. Sievers leads to the molecular mechanisms of apoptosis and their potential reversibility presented by J. Holtz.

All contributions presented at this workshop will help one to understand the complex mechanisms of the heart failure syndrome and, finally, make a step forward toward improved management of heart failure patients.

Basel, March 2000   *Prof. P. Buser*

Table of Contents

Chapter 1

The heart failure syndrome: new insights – from receptors to molecular biology

W. Schillinger and G. Hasenfuss

■ Introduction

During the last decade considerable advances in our understanding and management of heart failure have been made. However, with increasing life expectancy and decreasing mortality of acute myocardial infarction and other conditions that may cause heart failure, the incidence, prevalence, mortality, and economic costs of the disease are steadily increasing. The overall prevalence of congestive heart failure (CHF) is 1 to 2% in middle-aged and older adults, reaching 2 to 3% in patients older than age 65 years, and is 5 to 10% in patients beyond age 75 years [76]. Survival of patients suffering from heart failure depends of the duration and severity of the disease, on gender, as well as on therapeutic strategies. In the Framingham study, the overall 5-year survival rates were 25% in men and 38% in women [36]. In recent clinical trials with selected patients under state-of-the-art medical therapy, 1 year mortality ranged between 35% in patients with severe congestive heart failure (NYHA IV) in the Consensus trial [10] to 9% and 12% in patients with moderate CHF (NYHA II–III) in the second Vasodilator Heart Failure Trial [9] and the Studies of Left Ventricular Dysfunction (SOLVD) trial [66]. Mechanisms of death include sudden death in about 40%, worsening of heart failure in about 40%, and other factors in 20% of the patients.

■ Etiology of heart failure

Human heart failure has many underlying causes, the frequencies of which have changed considerably during the last decades. At present, the leading cause is coronary heart disease which accounted for 67% of CHF cases in the 1980s according to the Framingham heart study [36]. Most of these patients also had a history of arterial hypertension (57%). Valvular heart disease underlies failure in about 10% of the patients, and 20% of heart failure cases are attributable to primary myocardial diseases, of which dilated cardiomyopathy predominates. Regardless of the original cardiac abnormality, however, the advanced heart failure syndrome presents a complex picture including disturbed myocardial function, ventricular remodeling, altered hemodynamics, neurohumoral activation, cytokine overexpression, as well as vascular and endothelial dysfunction.

■ Neurohumoral and cytokine activation

Independent from the etiology of heart failure, activation of the neurohumoral and the cytokine system seems to play a critical role for the prognosis in CHF [22, 69, 70]. Activation of the neurohumoral systems occurs stepwise and organ specific as a consequence of altered organ perfusion (Fig. 1). It was shown recently that increased cardiac adrenergic drive precedes generalized sympathetic activation in patients with mild CHF [61]. This results from increased norepinephrine release and decreased norepinephrine reuptake and seems to be associated with early attenuation of cardiac and arterial baroreceptor control of sympathetic tone [15, 25]. Similarly, atrial natriuretic peptide is activated early in heart failure, and it was shown that atrial natriuretic peptide is elevated in asymptomatic patients with left ventricular dysfunction [21]. Although activation of local renin-angiotensin systems may occur early, plasma renin activity and vasopressin release are only increased in patients with symptomatic heart failure [21]. It is generally believed that neurohumoral and cytokine activation cause further damage to the failing heart like a vicious circle.

Recent studies have in particular identified the importance of cytokines as mediators of disease progression by mechanisms including necrotic and/or apoptotic myocyte cell death, myocardial fibrosis, and depression of myocardial function [for review see 65]. The influence of the vasoconstric-

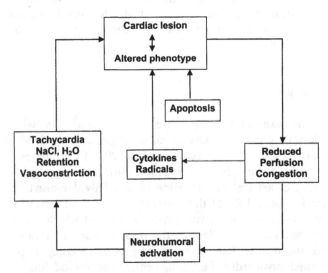

Fig. 1. Description of the pathophysiology of human heart failure as a vicius circle

tor peptide cytokine, endothelin, has been extensively investigated. Both mature endothelin-1 and its precursor, big endothelin-1, are increased in the peripheral circulation in relation to the hemodynamic and functional severity of heart failure, and plasma levels of big endothelin-1 are correlated with the prognosis of patients with heart failure [51]. Similarly, circulating levels of tumor necrosis factor (TNF)a, of TNF receptors, and of interleukin-6 are increased and positively related to the severity of heart failure [69]. TNF is expressed in the failing but not in the nonfailing human heart, whereas TNF receptors (TNFR1 and TNFR2) are expressed in failing and nonfailing myocardium [70].

It was recently shown that patients with chronic heart failure and peripheral edema exhibit increased endotoxin serum concentrations which were associated with increased concentrations of several cytokines including TNF [50]. The authors suggested that during edematous periods bacteria or endotoxin itself may translocate and trigger immune activation.

If TNF is of pathophysiological relevance in human heart failure, cytokine elimination or antagonism should be beneficial in those patients. This hypothesis is indeed supported by a recent safety and efficacy study of a soluble TNF receptor which binds and inhibits TNF. It was shown that intravenous application is safe and well tolerated in patients with NYHA class III heart failure and that this TNF receptor lowers levels of biologically active TNF and leads to improvement in the functional status of patients with heart failure [13].

■ Nitric oxide (NO)

There is considerable evidence that NO exhibits various effects on the myocardium. It may be involved in the induction of apoptosis, and may have direct cytotoxic effects. In addition, NO was shown to influence myocardial contraction. In the failing human heart, inducible NO synthase is expressed [35], resulting in increased cardiac NO activity. The latter was shown to increase rate of relaxation and to attenuate the positive inotropic effect of β-adrenoceptor stimulation [14]. These observations are supported by findings of Hare at al. that NO inhibits the positive inotropic response to β-adrenergic stimulation in humans with left ventricular dysfunction in vivo [28]. The functional importance of NO is further supported by recent clinical observations that exogenous NO and the stimulated release of NO from the endothelium modulates left ventricular function in humans [52, 53].

■ Myocardial alterations

At the level of the myocardium characteristic functional, biochemical, and molecular alterations occurring in end-stage heart failure have been described. Alterations occur at the level of the myocytes and the extracellular

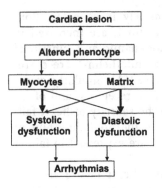

Fig. 2. Alterations at the level of the myocardium in human heart failure

matrix (Fig. 2). Functional studies in isolated muscle strip preparations showed that frequency potentiation of contractile force which is an important mechanism to regulate performance of the nonfailing heart is blunted in failing human myocardium [19, 26, 47]. This finding has been confirmed in clinical studies showing depressed frequency potentiation of hemodynamic parameters of myocardial performance [17, 30]. The term force-frequency relation generally is used to describe the relation between stimulation rate and developed force of the myocardium which represents the amplitude between diastolic force and peak systolic force. Accordingly, alterations of force-potentiation of myocardial function in failing human myocardium may result from altered systolic or altered diastolic function or from both.

Functional and subcellular alterations

There is accumulating evidence that an altered force-frequency relation results from disturbed calcium homeostasis. To study this, intracellular calcium transients have been evaluated using the photoprotein aequorin [55]. As is shown in Fig. 3, the frequency-dependent increase in isometric force observed in nonfailing human myocardium is associated with a parallel increase in aequorin light signal indicating an increase in the calcium transient. In contrast, inversion of the force-frequency relation is associated with a frequency-dependent decline of the calcium transient indicating decreased calcium release from the sarcoplasmic reticulum at higher stimulation rates in the failing human heart. This in turn may result from altered calcium-induced calcium release despite normal calcium load of the sarcoplasmic reticulum (SR) or from alterations in the SR calcium content.

To investigate these possibilities, post-rest potentiation and rapid cooling contractures have been measured in nonfailing and failing human myocardium [55, 57]: Fig. 4 shows post-rest potentiation measurements. When stimulation is stopped for a defined period of time, calcium is eliminated from the cytosol predominantly by calcium uptake into the SR and by calcium elimination across the sarcolemma by the Na^+-Ca^{2+} exchanger. Force

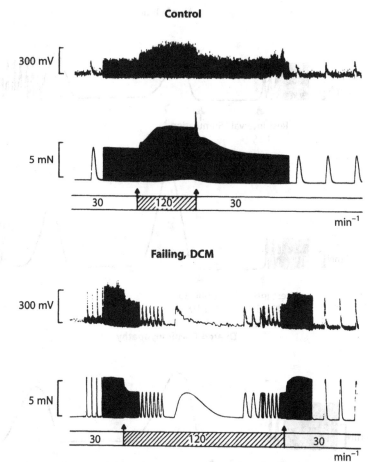

Fig. 3. Original recordings of aequorin light transients and isometric force signals in muscle strips from a nonfailing (control) and a failing human heart with dilated cardiomyopathy (DCM). In both experiments, stimulation frequency was changed from 30 min^{-1} to 120 min^{-1} and aequorin light (upper panels) and isometric force (lower panels) were recorded. Reproduced with permission from Pieske et al. (55)

development upon restimulation thus depends on the activity of these two transport mechanisms. As is obvious from the upper part of Fig. 4, post-rest potentiation of isometric force occurs in the nonfailing human myocardium indicating dominance of SR calcium uptake over transsarcolemmal calcium elimination. In contrast in a muscle strip from a failing human heart (lower 2 tracings) post-rest potentiation of force is attenuated after a rest period of 10 seconds and even converted to rest decay after a period of 120 seconds. This indicates increased transsarcolemmal calcium elimination relative to SR calcium uptake during the rest interval in the failing compared to the nonfailing myocardium. Disturbed sarcoplasmic reticulum calcium handling as a dominant cause for the altered force-fre-

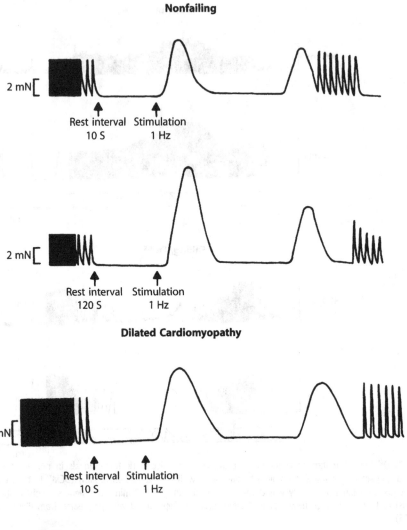

Nonfailing

Dilated Cardiomyopathy

Fig. 4. Influence of rest intervals on post-rest contraction. Original recordings of post-rest behavior in a muscle strip preparation from a nonfailing heart (top) and an end-stage failing heart (bottom). Rest intervals were 10 s and 120 s. Basal stimulation frequency was 1 Hz. Reproduced with permission from Pieske et al. (57)

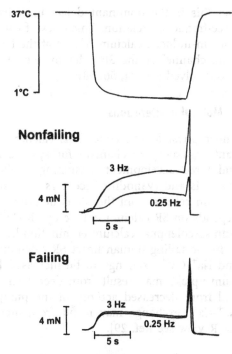

Fig. 5. Original recordings of isometric force during rapid cooling contractures in muscle strips from a nonfailing human heart (middle panel) and from an end-stage failing heart with idiopathic dilated cardiomyopathy (lower panel). Following steady-state stimulation at 0.25 Hz the temperature of the organ bath is rapidly decreased from 37 °C to 1 °C (upper panel) which results in complete SR calcium release and development of a contracture. Rewarming results in a rapid increase in force due to changes in calcium sensitivity followed by complete relaxation of the muscle. Thereafter, stimulation rate was increased to 3.0 Hz and the rapid cooling procedure was repeated during steady-state force development. Cross-sectional areas of muscle strips were 0.28 mm^2 (nonfailing) and 0.24 mm^2 (failing)

quency relation was also suggested from rapid cooling contracture measurements. This technique is based on the fact that rapid cooling (within 1 ms) of a muscle strip results in instantaneous release of all calcium stored in the SR with subsequent activation of contractile proteins and development of a contracture. Accordingly, development of a contracture following rapid cooling of a muscle strip preparation is an index of the calcium content of the sarcoplasmic reticulum. There is a pronounced increase in cooling contracture with increasing steady-state stimulation rates of twitches preceeding the rapid cooling procedure in nonfailing myocardium (middle panel of Fig. 5). The frequency-dependent increase in cooling contracture is blunted in the failing human heart (lower panel of Fig. 5).

The alterations of post-rest potentiations and rapid cooling contractures observed in the failing human myocardium strongly suggest that sarcoplasmic reticulum calcium loading is disturbed in the failing human heart and that this is the dominant defect underlying blunting or inversion of the force-frequency relation. This does of course not exclude that alterations in calcium-induced calcium release at the level of the sarcolemmal L-type calcium channel or the SR calcium release channel (ryanodine receptor) are also involved [11, 24, 56, 58].

Molecular alterations

Under physiological conditions calcium release from the SR is the dominant regulatory mechanism for systolic activation of contractile proteins and force development. Assuming unaltered function of L-type calcium channels and ryanodine receptors and unaltered interaction between both, calcium release from the SR is determined by SR calcium load. The latter depends on SR calcium uptake by SR Ca^{2+}-ATPase which is in competition with sarcolemmal calcium elimination by the Na^+-Ca^{2+} exchanger.

In the failing human heart SR calcium uptake was shown to be reduced and Na^+-Ca^{2+} exchange to be increased [32, 39, 60, 64]. Reduced SR calcium uptake may result from decreased SR calcium ATPase protein levels and from decreased activity of the pump [44, 62, 64, 67], and increased Na^+-Ca^{2+} exchange may result from increased protein levels [20, 67, and for Review see Ref. 29].

Relationship between frequency-dependence of systolic and diastolic function and protein levels of SR Ca^{2+}-ATPase and Na^+-Ca^{2+} exchanger

The relevance of SR Ca^{2+}-ATPase and Na^+-Ca^{2+} exchanger protein levels on systolic and diastolic function was recently evaluated in a study which was primarily designed to test the hypothesis that in end-stage failing human hearts diastolic function would greatly depend on protein levels of the Na^+-Ca^{2+} exchanger [33]. Endstage failing hearts were divided into three groups according to their diastolic function. As shown in Fig. 6, hearts without an increase in diastolic force upon a rise of the stimulation rate represent group I. In group II hearts there was a moderate increase and in group III hearts there was a pronounced increase in diastolic force with increasing stimulation rate. As shown in Fig. 7, in hearts with normal diastolic function Na^+-Ca^{2+} exchanger protein levels were increased compared to nonfailing human myocardium and SERCA protein levels were not significantly reduced. Thus the capacity for calcium elimination is high. In contrast, in hearts with severely compromised diastolic function, Na^+-Ca^{2+} exchanger was not upregulated and SERCA protein levels were significantly depressed compared to nonfailing myocardium. However, in all failing hearts, the ratio of Na^+-Ca^{2+}-exchanger to SERCA was significantly increased compared to nonfailing hearts. This alteration favors decreased SR calcium load and thus decreased calcium available for release and systolic activation of contractile proteins in the failing human heart and causes systolic dysfunction and alteration of the force-frequency relation (Fig. 8).

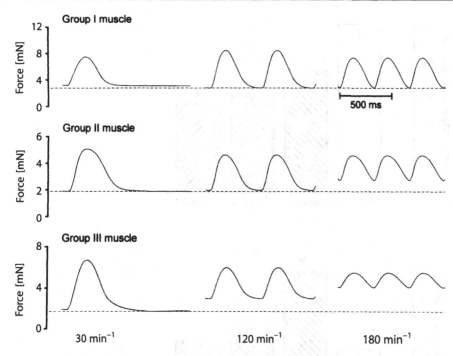

Fig. 6. Original recordings of isometrically contracting failing human myocardium. Upper panel: Muscle strip representative for group I hearts showing a slight decrease of diastolic force at 120 versus 30 min^{-1} (cross-sectional area was 0.25 mm^2). Middle panel: Muscle strip representative for group II hearts showing a moderate increase in diastolic force from 30 to 180 min^{-1} (cross-sectional area was 0.16 mm^2). Lower panel: Muscles strip representative for group III hearts exhibiting a pronounced rise of diastolic force from 30 to 120 and 180 min^{-1} (cross-sectional area was 0.16 mm^2)

Besides alteration in protein expression of SR Ca^{2+}-ATPase and Na^+-Ca^{2+} exchanger, levels of protein phosphorylation are critically important for transport activity into the SR or across the sarcolemma. Phosphorylation of phospholamban, the regulatory protein of SR Ca^{2+}-ATPase, by protein kinase A and calcium/calmodulin-dependent protein kinase results in increased calcium sensitivity and activity of the pump [37, 74]. The β-adrenoceptor-adenylyl cyclase system is downregulated in the failing human heart which may result in decreased protein kinase A activity, and therefore reduced phosphorylation of phospholamban. This may contribute to decreased sarcoplasmic reticulum calcium transport, and altered force-frequency relation (see below).

Contractile proteins

Although myosin content may be decreased by about 20% due to replacement by connective tissue [31], maximum calcium activated force was suggested to be similar in failing and nonfailing human myocardium [18, 23].

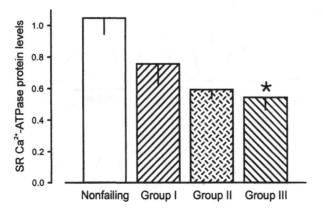

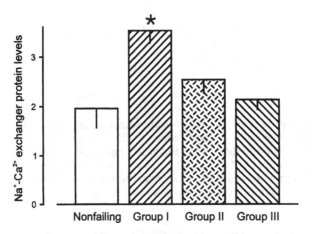

Fig. 7. Graph showing protein levels of SERCA and Na$^+$-Ca^{2+} exchanger in failing and nonfaiing human myocardium. Protein levels are normalized to calsequestrin protein levels. * = p < 0.05 vs. nonfailing

This may be because force-time integral production of the individual cross-bridge cycle is increased in the failing heart, associated with reduced myo-fibrillar ATPase activity [1, 31]. Previous studies suggested that unlike the situation in small mammals alteration of crossbridge function may not be related to a myosin isoform shift, because it was observed that the β-myo-sin heavy chain isoform predominates in the left ventricle of nonfailing and failing human hearts [43]. This is in contrast to more recent studies in which at the level of mRNA ventricular expression of the α-myosin heavy chain isoform was observed in nonfailing hearts, which was decreased in failing human hearts [40, 49]. Alternatively to a myosin isoform shift, the alteration in crossbridge function may, however, be related to changes in troponin T isoforms or alterations in myosin light chains [2, 41]. Contro-versy exists regarding alteration of myofilament calcium sensitivity as mea-

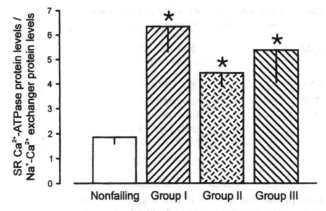

Fig. 8. Ratio of Na^+-Ca^{2+} exchanger to SERCA protein levels. Increased ratio may indicate a shift from sarcoplasmic reticulum to transsarcolemmal calcium elimination from the cytosol which may be associated with cellular loss of calcium for activation of contractile proteins. $* = p < 0.05$ vs. nonfailing

sured in myofibrillar preparations which was suggested to be unchanged [11, 27] or increased [63]. Wolff et al. suggested that calcium sensitivity is increased in failing myocardium from hearts with dilated cardiomyopathy which may be due in part to a reduction of protein kinase A-dependent phosphorylation of myofibrillar regulatory proteins [75].

Sarcolemmal receptors

Bristow et al. were the first to demonstrate that in end-stage heart failure the number of β-adrenoceptors and the inotropic response to isoproterenol is reduced [7]. β-adrenoceptor downregulation was shown to be in direct relation to the severity of ventricular dysfunction, to be independent from the etiology of heart failure, and to result from a decreased density of β1-adrenoceptors, whereas β2-adrenoceptor density remains unchanged [8]. The β1-adrenoceptor downregulation seems to result predominantly from decreased de novo synthesis, as indicated by decreased β1-adrenoceptor mRNA levels [6, 72]. In addition, increased breakdown may be involved. Downregulation seems to be the consequence of increased and prolonged catecholamine exposure of the failing myocardium [for review, see 8]. In addition to downregulation (loss of receptors), desensitization (loss of response) of the β-adrenoceptor occurs after short-term exposure catecholamines. Desensitization is initiated by phosphorylation of the occupied receptors by β-adrenoceptor kinase (homologous desensitization) and by PKA (heterologous desensitization). Phosphorylation is thought to induce uncoupling of the β-adrenoceptor from the stimulatory Gs protein [48]. Expression of β-adrenoceptor kinase has recently been shown to be increased in the failing human heart, which may result in augmented homologous desensitization [72].

Table 1. Alterations of receptors in human heart failure

β_1-AR ↓	Bristow 1982 (7)
β_2-AR →	Böhm 1988 (4)
	Brodde 1991 (8)
α-AR ↑	Vago 1989 (73)
AT$_1$-R ↓	Haywood 1997 (34)
AT$_2$-R (↑), →, (↓)	Asano 1997 (3)
	Regitz-Zagrosek (59)
	Tsutsumi 1998 (71)
ET$_A$-R ↑	Pieske 1999 (54)
ET$_B$-R →	

β_1-AR β_1 adrenoceptor; α-AR α adrenoceptor; AT$_1$-R and AT$_2$-R angiotensin receptors subtype 1 and subtype 2; ET$_A$-R and ET$_B$-R endothelin receptor subtypes

In addition to downregulation and desensitization of β1-adrenoceptor in the failing human heart, the decreased inotropic response to β-adrenoceptor stimulators is related to increased levels of the inhibitory G protein in this setting [5, 16]. In contrast, the stimulating Gs protein, as well as the catalytic subunit of adenylyl cyclase, seem to be unaltered in human heart failure [16]. As may be expected from the described alterations in the β-adrenoceptor adenylyl cyclase system, reduced basal and isoprenaline-stimulated cAMP levels in failing human myocardium were reported [12]; however, others found that total cAMP levels and activity of PKA are unchanged during basal conditions in the failing human heart [46].

Besides the β-adrenoceptor-system, alterations have been observed in angiotensin receptors, in endothelin receptors as well as in alpha receptor of the myocardium (Table 1).

Extracellular matrix

Quantitative and qualitative alterations have been observed in extracellular matrix proteins in failing human myocardium (Table 2). These include in-

Table 2. Extracellular matrix in human heart failure

Connective tissue content ↑	Hasenfuss 1992 (31)
Collagen composition	
type I/type III ↑	Marijianowski 1995 (42)
type VI ↑	Mollnau 1995 (45)
Matrix Metalloproteinases	
MMP 3 ↑	Spinale 1998 (68)
MMP 9 ↑	
TIMPs ↓	Li 1998 (38)

creased connective tissue content and altered collagene composition. More recently, increased expression of matrix metalloproteinases and decreased expression of tissue inhibitors of metalloproteinases have been discribed in the failing human heart. The increased activity of matrix metalloproteinases may result in myocyte slippage and ventricular dilatation, increased stiffness, and impaired diastolic function (Table 2).

■ Summary

Congestive heart failure is a complex syndrome which includes disturbed myocardial function and neurohumoral and cytokine activation. In end-stage failure, alteration of extracellular matrix as well as alteration of myocyte phenotype contribute to disturbed myocardial function. At the level of the myocyte, altered calcium homeostasis seems to play a dominant role. Recent progress in molecular analyses of the pathophysiological processes will allow the development molecular strategies for the therapy of human heart failure.

■ References

1. Alpert NR, Gordon MS (1962) Myofibrillar adenosine triphosphatase activity in congestive heart failure. Am J Physiol 202:940–946
2. Anderson PA, Malouf NN, Oakeley AE, Pagani ED, Allen PD (1991) Troponin T isoform expression in humans. A comparison among normal and failing adult heart, fetal heart, and adult and fetal skeletal muscle. Circ Res 69:1226–1233
3. Asano K, Dutcher DL, Port JD, Minobe WA, Tremmel KD, Roden RL, Bohlmeyer TJ, Bush EW, Jenkin MJ, Abraham WT, Raynolds MV, Zisman LS, Perryman MB, Bristow MR (1997) Selective downregulation of the angiotensin II AT1-receptor subtype in failing human ventricular myocardium. Circulation 95:1193–1200
4. Bohm M, Diet F, Feiler G, Kembkes B, Kreuzer E, Weinhild C, Erdmann E (1988) Subsensitivity of the failing human heart to isoprenaline and milrinone is related to beta-adrenoceptor downregulation. J Cardiovasc Pharmacol 12:726–732
5. Bohm M, Larisch K, Erdmann E, Camps M, Jakobs K, Gierschik P (1991) Failure of [32P]ADP-ribosylation by pertussis toxin to determine Gi alpha content in membranes from various human tissues. Improved radioimmunological quantification using the 125I-labelled C-terminal decapeptide of retinal transducin. Biochem J 277:223–229
6. Bristow MR, Minobe WA, Raynolds MV, Port JD, Rasmussen R, Ray PE, Feldman AM (1993) Reduced beta 1 receptor messenger RNA abundance in the failing human heart. J Clin Invest 92:2737–2745
7. Bristow MR, Ginsburg R, Minobe W, Cubicciotti RS, Sageman WS, Lurie K, Billingham ME, Harrison DC, Stinson EB (1982) Decreased catecholamine sensitivity and beta-adrenergic-receptor density in failing human hearts. N Engl J Med 307:205–211
8. Brodde OE (1991) Beta 1- and beta 2-adrenoceptors in the human heart: properties, function, and alterations in chronic heart failure. Pharmacol Rev 43:203–242

9. Cohn JN, Johnson G, Ziesche S, Cobb F, Francis G, Tristani F, Smith R, Dunkman WB, Loeb H, Wong M et al (1991) A comparison of enalapril with hydralazine-isosorbide dinitrate in the treatment of chronic congestive heart failure. N Engl J Med 325:303–310

10. The CONSENSUS Trial Study Group (1987) Effects of enalapril on mortality in severe congestive heart failure. Results of the Cooperative North Scandinavian Enalapril Survival Study (CONSENSUS). N Engl J Med 316:1429–1435

11. D'Agnolo A, Luciani GB, Mazzucco A, Gallucci V, Salviati G (1992) Contactile properties and Ca^{2+} release activity of the sarcoplasmic reticulum in dilated cardiomyopathy. Circulation 85:518–525

12. Danielsen W, v der Leuyen H, Meyer W, Neumann J, Schmitz W, Scholz H, Starbatty J, Stein B, Doring V, Kalmar P (1989) Basal and isoprenaline-stimulated cAMP content in failing versus nonfailing human cardiac preparations. J Cardiovasc Pharmacol 14:171–173

13. Deswal A, Bozkurt B, Seta Y, Parilti-Eiswirth S, Hayes FA, Flosch C, Mann DL (1999) Safety and efficacy of a soluble P75 tumor necrosis factor receptor (Enbrel, etanercept) in patients with advanced heart failure. Circulation 99:3224–3226

14. Drexler H, Kästner S, Strobel A, Studer R, Brodde OE, Hasenfuss G (1998) Expression, activity and functional significance of endothelial and inducible nitric oxide synthase in the failing human heart. JACC 32:955–963

15. Eisenhofer G, Friberg P, Rundqvist B, Quyyumi AA, Lambert G, Kaye DM, Kopin IJ, Goldstein DS, Esler MD (1996) Cardiac sympathetic nerve function in congestive heart failure. Circulation 93:1667–1676

16. Feldman AM, Cates AE, Veazey WB, Hershberger RE, Bristow MR, Baughman KL, Baumgartner WA, Van Dop C (1988) Increase of the 40 000-mol wt pertussis toxin substrate (G protein) in the failing human heart. J Clin Invest 82:189–197

17. Feldman MD, Alderman JD, Aroesty JM, Royal HD, Ferguson JJ, Owen RM, Grossman W, McKay RG (1988) Depression of systolic and diastolic myocardial reverse during atrial pacing tachycardia in patients with dilated cardiomyopathy. J Clin Invest 82:1661–1669

18. Feldman MD, Copelas L, Gwathmey JK, Philips P, Warren SE, Schoen FJ, Grossman W, Morgan JP (1987) Deficient production of cyclic AMP: pharmacologic evidence of an important cause of contractile dysfunction in patients with end-stage heart failure. Circulation 75:331–339

19. Feldman MD, Gwathmey JK, Phillips P, Schoen F, Morgan JP (1988) Reversal of the force-frequency relationship in working myocardium from patients with end-stage heart failure. J Appl Cardiol 3:273–283

20. Flesch M, Schwinger RH, Schiffer F, Frank K, Sudkamp M, Kuhn-Regnier F, Arnold G, Bohm M (1996) Evidence for functional relevance of an enhanced expression of the Na^+-Ca^{2+} exchanger in failing human myocardium. Circulation 94:992–1002

21. Francis GS, Benedict C,, Johnstone DE, Kirlin PC, Nicklas J, Liang CS, Kubo SH, Rudin-Toretsky E, Yusuf S (1990) Comparison of neuroendocrine activation in patients with left ventricular dysfunction with and without congestive heart failure. A substudy of the Studies of Left Ventricular Dysfunction (SOLVD). Circulation 82:1724-1729

22. Francis GS, Cohn JN, Johnson G, Rector TS, Goldman S, Simon A (1993) Plasma norepinephrine, plasma renin activity, and congestive heart failure. Relations to survival and the effects of therapy in V-HeFT II. The V-HeFT VA Cooperative Studies Group. Circulation 87 (Suppl VI):40–48

23. Ginsburg R, Bristow MR, Billingham ME, Stinson EB, Schroeder JS, Harison DC (1983) Study of the normal and failing isolated human heart: decrease of failing heart to isoproterenol. Am Heart J 106:535–540

24. Gomez AM, Valdivia HH, Cheng H, Lederer MR, Santana LF, Cannell MB, McCune SA, Altschuld RA, Lederer WJ (1997) Defective excitation-contraction coupling in experimental cardiac hypertrophy and heart failure. Science 276:800–806
25. Grassi G, Saravelle G, Cattaneo BM, Lanfranchi A, Vailati S, Giannattasio C, Del Bo A, Sala C, Bolla GB, Pozzi M (1995) Sympathetic activation and loss of reflex sympathetic control in mild congestive heart failure. Circulation 92:3206–3211
26. Gwathmey JK, Slawsky MT, Hajjar RJ, Briggs GM, Morgan JP (1990) Role of intra-cellular calcium handling in force-interval relationships of human ventricular myocardium. J Clin Invest 85:1599–1613
27. Hajjar RJ, Gwathmey JK, Briggs GM, Morgan JP (1988) Differential effect of DPI 201-106 on the sensitivity of the myofilaments to Ca^{2+} in intact and skinned tra-beculae from control and myopathic human hearts. J Clin Invest 82:1578–1584
28. Hare JM, Loh E, Creager MA, Colucci WS (1995) Nitric oxide inhibits the positive inotropic response to beta-adrenergic stimulation in humans with left ventricular dysfunction. Circulation 92:2198–2203
29. Hasenfuss G (1998) Alterations of calcium-regulatory proteins in heart failure. Cardiovasc Res 37:279–289
30. Hasenfuss G, Holubarsch C, Hermann HP, Astheimer K, Pieske B, Just H (1994) Influence of the force-frequency relationship on haemodynamics and left ventri-cular function in patients with non-failing hearts and in patients with dilated car-diomyopathy. Eur Heart J 15:164–170
31. Hasenfuss G, Mulieri LA, Leavitt BJ, Allen PD, Haeberle JR, Alpert NR (1992) Al-teration of contractile function and excitation-contraction coupling in dilated car-diomyopathy. Circ Res 70:1225–1232
32. Hasenfuss G, Reinecke H, Studer R, Meyer M, Pieske B, Holtz J, Holubarsch C, Posival H, Just H, Drexler H (1994) Relation between myocardial function and ex-pression of sarcoplasmic reticulum Ca^{2+}-ATPase in failing and nonfailing human myocardium Circ Res 75:434–442
33. Hasenfuss G, Schillinger W, Lehnart SE, Preuss M, Pieske B, Maier LS, Prestle J, Minami K, Just H (1999) Relationship between Na^{+}-Ca^{2+} exchanger protein levels and diastolic function in failing human myocardium. Circulation 99:641–648
34. Haywood GA, Gullestad L, Katsuya T, Hutchinson HG, Pratt RE, Horiuchi M, Fowler MB (1997) AT1 and AT2 angiotensin receptor gene expression in human heart failure. Circulation 95:1201–1206
35. Haywood GA, Tsao PS, von der Leyen HE, Man MJ, Keeling PJ, Trindade PT, Lewis NP, Byrne CD, Rickenbacher PR, Bishopric NH, Cooke JP, McKenna WJ, Fowler MB (1996) Expression of inducible nitric oxide synthase in human heart failure. Circulation 93:1087–1094
36. Ho KK, Anderson KM, Kannel WB, Grossman W, Levy D (1993) Survival after the onset of congestive heart failure in Framingham Heart Study subjects. Circulation 88:107–115
37. Kranias EG, Garvey JL, Srivastava RD, Solaro RJ (1985) Phosphorylation and functional modifications of sarcoplasmic reticulum and myofibrils in isolated rab-bit hearts stimulated with isoprenaline. Biochem J 226:113–121
38. Li YY, Feldman AM, Sun Y, McTierman CF (1998) Differential expression of tis-sue inhibitors of metalloproteinase in the failing human heart. Circulation 98:1728–1734
39. Limas CJ, Olivari MT, Goldenberg IF, Levine TB, Benditt DG, Simon A (1987) Cal-cium uptake by cardiac sarcoplasmic reticulum in human dilated cardiomyopathy. Cardiovasc Res 21:601–605
40. Lowes BD, Minobe W, Abraham WT, Rizeq MN, Bohlmeyer TJ, Quaife RA, Roden RL, Dutcher DL, Robertson AD, Voelkel NF, Badesch DB, Groves BM, Gilbert EM,

Bristow MR (1997) Changes in gene expression in the intact human heart. Down-regulation of alpha-myosin heavy chain in hypertrophied, failing venctricular myocardium. J Clin Invest 100:2315–2324

41. Margossian SS, White HD, Caulfield JB, Norton P, Taylor S, Slayter HS (1992) Light chain 2 profile and activity of human ventricular myosin during dilated cardiomyopathie. Identification of a causal agent for impaired myocardial function. Circulation 85:1720–1733

42. Marijianowski MM, Teeling P, Mann J, Becker AE (1995) Dilated cardiomyopathy is associated with an increase in the type I/type III collagen ratio: a quantitative assessment. J Am Coll Cardiol 25:1263–1272

43. Mercadier JJ, Bouveret P, Gorza L, Schiaffino S, Clark WA, Zak R, Swynghedauw B, Schwartz K (1983) Myosin isoenzymes in normal and hypertrophied human ventricular myocardium. Circ Res 53:52–62

44. Meyer M, Schillinger W, Pieske B, Holubarsch C, Heilmann C, Posival H, Kuwajima G, Mikoshiba K, Just H, Hasenfuss G (1995) Alterations of sarcoplasmic reticulum proteins in failing human dilated cardiomyopathy. Circulation 92:778–784

45. Mollnau H, Munkel B, Schaper J (1995) Collagen VI in the extracellular matrix of normal and failing human myocardium. Herz 20:89–94

46. Morgan JP, Emy RE, Allen PD, Grossman W, Gwathmey JK (1990) Abnormal intracellular calcium handling, a major cause of systolic and diastolic dysfunction in ventricular myocardium from patients with heart failure. Circulation 81 (Suppl III):21–32

47. Mulieri LA, Hasenfuss G, Leavitt B, Allen PD, Alpert NR (1992) Altered myocardial force-frequency relation in human heart failure. Circulation 85:1743–1750

48. Muntz KH, Zhao M, Miller JC (1994) Downregulation of myocardial beta-adrenergic receptors. Receptor subtype selectivity. Circ Res 74:369–375

49. Nakao K, Minobe W, Roden R, Bristow MR, Leinwand LA (1997) Myosin heavy chain gene expression in human heart failure. J Clin Invest 100:2362–2370

50. Niebeauer J, Volk HD, Kemp M, Dominguez M, Schumann RR, Rauchhaus M, Pool-Wilson PA, Coats AJ, Anker SD (1999) Endotoxin and immune activation in chronic heart failure: a prospective cohort study. Lancet 353:1838–1842

51. Pacher R, Stanek B, Hulsmann M, Koller-Strametz J, Berger R, Schuller M, Hartter E, Orgris E, Frey B, heinz G, Maurer G (1996) Prognostic impact of big endothelin-1 plasma concentrations compared with invasive hemodynamic evaluation in severe heart failure. J Am Coll Cardiol 27:633–641

52. Paulus WJ, Vantrimpont PJ, Shah AM (1994) Acute effects of nitric oxide on left ventricular relaxation and diastolic distensibility in humans by hastening left ventricular relaxation Circulation 89:2070–2078

53. Paulus WJ, Vantrimpont PJ, Shah AM (1995) Paracrine coronary endothelial control of left ventricular function in humans. Circulation 92:2119–2126

54. Pieske B, Beyermann B, Breu V, Loffler BM, Schlotthauer K, Maier LS, Schmidt-Schweda S, Just H, Hasenfuss G (1999) Functional effects of endothelin and regulation of endothelin receptors in isolated human nonfailing and failing myocardium. Circulation 99:1802–1809

55. Pieske B, Kretschmann B, Meyer M, Holubarsch C, Weirich J, Posival H, Minami K, Just H, Hasenfuss G (1995) Alterations in intracellular calcium handling associated with the inverse force-frequency relation in human dilated cardiomyopathy. Circulation 92:1169–1178

56. Pieske B, Maier LS, Bers D, Hasenfuss G (1999) Ca^{2+} handling and sarcoplasmic reticulum Ca^{2+} content in isolated failing and nonfailing human myocardium. Circ Res 85:38–46

57. Pieske B, Sutterlin M, Schmidt-Schweda S, Minami K, Meyer M, Olschewski M, Holubarsch C, Just H, Hasenfuss G (1996) Diminished post-rest potentiation of

contractile force in human dilated cardiomyopathie. Functional evidence for alterations in intracellular Ca^{2+} handling. J Clin Invest 98:764–776

58. Piot C, Lemaire S, Albat B, Seguin J, Nargeot J, Richard S (1996) High frequency-induced upregulation of human cardiac calcium currents. Circulation 93:128

59. Regitz-Zagrosek V, Fielitz J, Dreysse R, Hildebrandt AG, Fleck E (1997) Angiotensin receptor type 1 mRNA in human right ventricular endomyocardial biopsies: downregulation in heart failure. Cardiovasc Res 35:99–105

60. Reinecke H, Studer R, Vetter R, Holtz J, Drexler H (1996) Cardiac Na^2/Ca^{2+} exchange activity in patients with end-stage heart failure. Cardiovasc Res 31:48–54

61. Rundqvist B, Elam M, Bergmann-Sverrisdottir Y, Eisenhofer G, Friberg P (1997) Increased cardiac adrenergic drive precedes generalized sympathetic activation in human heart failure. Circulation 95:169–175

62. Schillinger W, Meyer M, Kuwajima G, Katsuhiko M, Just H, Hasenfuss G (1996) Unaltered ryanodine receptor protein levels in ischemic cardiomyopathy. Mol Cell Biochem 160/161:297–302

63. Schwinger RH, Bohm M, Koch A, Schmidt U, Morano I, Eissner HJ, Uberfuhr P, Reichart B, Erdmann E (1994) The failing human heart is unable to use the Frank-Starling mechanism. Circ Res 74:959–969

64. Schwinger RH, Bohm M, Schmidt U, Karczweski P, Bavendiek U, Flesch M, Krause EG, Erdmann E (1995) Unchanged protein levels of SERCA II and phospholamban but reduced Ca^{2+} uptake and Ca^{2+}-ATPase of cardiac sarcoplasmic reticulum from dilated cardiomyopathy patients compared with patients with non-failing hearts. Circulation 92:3220–3228

65. Shan K, Kurrelmeyer K, Seta Y, Wang F, Dibbs Z, Deswal A, Lee-Jackson D, Mann DL (1997) The role of cytokines in disease progression in heart failure. Curr Opin Cardiol 12:218–223

66. The SOLVD Investigators (1991) Effect of enalapril on survival in patients with reduced left ventricular ejection fractions and congestive heart failure. N Engl J Med 325:293–302

67. Studer R, Reinecke H, Bilger J, Eschenhagen T, Bohm M, Hasenfuss G, Just H, Holtz J, Drexler H (1994) Gene expression of the cardiac Na^+-Ca^{2+} exchanger in end-stage human heart failure. Circ Res 75:443–453

68. Spinale FG, Cocker ML, Thomas CV, Walker JD, Mukherjee R, Hebbar L (1998) Time-dependent changes in matrix metalloproteinase activity and expression during the progression of congestive heart failure: relation to ventricular and myocyte function. Circ Res 82:482–495

69. Torre-Amione G, Kapadia S, Benedict C, Oral H, Young JB, Mann DL (1996) Proinflammatory cytokine levels in patients with depressed left ventricular ejection fraction: a report from the Studies of Left Ventricular Dysfunction (SOLVD). J Am Coll Cardiol 27:1201–1206

70. Torre-Amione G, Kapadia S, Lee J, Durand JB, Bies RD, Young JB, Mann DL (1996) Tumor necrosis factor-alpha and tumor necrosis factor receptors in the failing human heart. Circulation 93:704–711

71. Tsutsumi Y, Matsubara H, Ohkubo N, Mori Y, Nozawa Y, Murasawa S, Kijima K, Maruyama K, Masaki H, Moriguchi Y, Shibasaki Y, Kamihata H, Inada M, Iwasaka T (1998) Antiotensin II type 2 receptor is upregulated in human heart with interstitial fibrosis, and cardiac fibroblasts are the major cell type for its expression. Circ Res 83:1035–1046

72. Ungerer M, Bohm M, Elce JS, Erdmann E, Lohse MJ (1993) Altered expression of beta-adrenergic receptor kinase and beta 1-adrenergic receptors in the failing human heart. Circulation 87:454–463

73. Vago T, Bevilacqua M, Norbiato G, Baldi G, Chabat E, Bertora P, Baroldi G, Accinni R (1989) Identification of alpha 1-adrenergic receptors on sarcolemma from

normal subjects and patients with idiopathic dilated cardiomyopathy: characteristics and linkage to GTP-binding protein. Circ Res 64:474–481
74. Voss J, Jones LR, Thomas DD (1994) The physical mechanism of calcium pump regulation in the heart. Biophysical Journal 67:190–196
75. Wolff MR, Buck SH, Stoker SW, Greaser ML, Mentzer RM (1996) Myofibrillar calcium sensitivity of isometric tension is increased in human dilated cardiomyopathies: role of altered beta-adrenergically mediated protein phosphorylation. J Clin Invest 98:167–176
76. Yamani M, Massie BM (1993) Congestive heart failure: insights from epidemiology, implications for treatment. Mayo Clin Proc 68:1214–1218

Author's address:

Prof. Dr. Gerd Hasenfuss
Zentrum Innere Medizin
Abteilung Kardiologie und Pneumologie, Universität Göttingen
Robert-Koch-Str. 40
37075 Göttingen, Germany
Phone: 011 49-551-39 63 51
E-mail: hasenfus@med.uni-goettingen.de

CHAPTER **2** **End stage heart failure –
options for medical treatment
and beyond**

P. A. POOLE-WILSON

▤ Introduction

Heart failure is a common disease which is becoming more common. Until ten years ago heart failure was the Cinderella of cardiology overshadowed by the lustre and glitter of its two sisters intervention and technology. That has changed. The two main reasons have been, first, appreciation of the clinical importance of heart failure as a major health care problem and, second, the excitement generated by the introduction of new treatments, advances in biology and availability of surgical options such as transplantation.

Heart failure has a prevalence of between 1 and 3% of the population and an incidence of approximately 1% [6]. 50% of patients with heart failure die within five years (Table 1). Heart failure is a major factor contributing to the occupation of about 5% of hospital beds. Of those admitted to the hospital 40% will be re-admitted in one year and the annual mortality is approximately 40%. In Western countries the condition consumes between 1 and 2% of the overall health budget.

There are two dominant reasons for the emergence of heart failure as such an important entity. The improved treatment of myocardial infarction and the reduction in case mortality has increased the number of persons who are alive but have a damaged heart; these patients go on to develop heart failure. Alterations in demography are occurring in most Western

Table 1. Prognosis of heart failure

▨ Overall mortality	25% at 2 years and 50% at 5 years
▨ NYHA class IV	50% at 1 year
▨ NYHA class III	30% at 1 year
▨ Predictors:	1. Extent of ventricular damage LVEF, heart size, haemodynamics, NYHA class, symptoms, signs
	2. Myocardial reserve Peak VO_2, NYHA class, symptoms
	3. Metabolic response Cachexia, hormones, cytokines, symptoms

countries with an increase in the proportion of elderly persons in the population. Heart failure and indeed coronary heart disease are diseases of the elderly. Thus, although there may be an anticipated age specific reduction in the mortality from coronary heart disease over the next twenty years, total mortality and morbidity from coronary heart disease will increase. Underlying this argument is the fact that most treatments for heart failure, other than transplantation, alleviate symptoms and prolong mortality but do not cure the entity or prevent the continuing ravages of the commonest cause (80%) namely coronary heart disease. The treatments merely delay the onset of worsening symptoms.

■ Definitions of severity

Heart failure is a clinical syndrome easily recognised by doctors and characterised by a particular pattern of symptoms, physical signs and body responses [19–21]. The commonest symptoms are fatigue, tiredness and shortness of breath. The severity of heart failure clinically is classified according to the New York Heart Association Classification. In broad terms the severity of heart failure assessed using this classification does relate to the severity of symptoms and also to mortality. The relationship with mortality, however, is poor. For example in three recent trials of beta blockers in heart failure (CIBIS II [4], MERIT [13], BEST) the annual mortality in those classified as NYHA Class III was 12.0%, 13.2% and 15.7% per annum. Such a huge variation indicates a lack of accuracy and reproducibility between doctors in using this classification. The key problems are the difficulty in taking a clinical history, variation of symptoms with time and a lack of understanding of the underlying causes of symptoms particularly in an individual patient (Table 2).

There are many predictors of outcome in heart failure (Table 1). These in general can be classified as relating to the extent of damage to the heart, the reserve function of the heart and the body responses. Thus, the oft

Table 2. Origin of symptoms in chronic heart failure

■ Lungs	Increased stiffness due to raised venous pressure and lymphatic distension
	Increased left atrial pressure
	Increased physiological dead space
	Increased respiratory rate
	Weakness of diaphragm
■ Circulation	Reduced blood flow to skeletal muscle
	Increased production of metabolites
	Altered response to metabolites
■ Skeletal muscle	Rest atrophy
	Ischemic atrophy
	Activation of ergoreceptors

stated aphorism that a big heart is a bad heart is a general truth, although heart failure can frequently be associated with a small heart and occasionally large hearts are compatible with a long life of reasonable quality. The ejection fraction which is much used for classification of heart failure in general measures the size of the ventricle rather than being a measure of function. The ejection fraction is determined largely by the denominator, the end-diastolic volume. The maximum oxygen consumption is a satisfactory measure of myocardial reserve because its relation to cardiac output is described by the Fick equation. Many metabolic markers including simple measurements such as serum sodium or complex measurements such as those of cytokines and immune activation also predict outcome. In severe heart failure these three variables (ejection fraction, oxygen consumption and serum sodium) are the most useful predictors of outcome [16].

The key difficulty for the physician is the definition and diagnosis of severe heart failure. A simple view would be that severe heart failure is present when a patient is in NYHA class III or IV. But patients in class III are often misclassified. With regard to the evaluation of new treatments in severe heart failure it is probably more appropriate to focus on class IV patients. These patients are usually short of breath at rest and virtually bedridden. The formal definition of class IV is "Patients with cardiac disease resulting in inability to carry on any physical activity without discomfort. Symptoms of heart failure or the anginal syndrome may be present even at rest. If any physical activity is undertaken, discomfort is increased" [7].

■ Medical treatment

The objectives of treatment in heart failure are no different to any other medical condition, namely to reduce symptoms and prolong life (Table 3). There are no other reasons for treatment. Prevention is not a key issue because chronic disease is already established and by definition cannot be

Table 3. Objektives of treatment in chronic heart failure

■ Prevention	Myocardial damage	Occurrence
		Progression of damage
		Further damaging episodes
	Reoccurrence	Symptoms
		Fluid accumulation
		Hospitalisation
■ Relief of symptoms and signs	Eliminate oedema and fluid retention	
	Increase exercise capacity	
	Reduce fatigue and breathlessness	
■ Prognosis	Reduce mortality	

Table 4. Severe heart failure: augmentation of standard treatment for heart failure

Intravenous drugs	Diuretics or combination of diuretics
	Nitrates
	Positive inotropes – dopamine/dobutamine
Fluid control	Haemofiltration
	Peritoneal dialysis or haemodialysis
Devices	ICD or pacing
	Intraaortic balloon pump
	Ventricular assist device
	Total artificial heart
Surgery	CABG for "hibernation"
	Valve surgery
	Cardiomyoplasty
	Volume reduction
	Transplantation

Table 5. Drugs in the treatment of chronic heart failure

Diuretics	Loop, thiazide, K^+ sparing diuretics, spironolactone or combination	
ACE inhibitors		
Beta-blockers		
Digoxin		
Aspirin, statins, anticoagulants, angiotensin II receptor inhibitors		
Vasodilators (nitrates, hydralazine), intermittent IV inotropes		
Others	Calcium antagonists	Salbutamol
	Aminophylline	Antiarrhythmics

prevented. The medical treatment of heart failure and of severe heart failure is shown in Tables 4, 5 and 6. There have been many approaches to the management of heart failure. Some have involved detailed measurements of haemodynamics. A more practical view is to use diuretics in order to control the fluid volumes within the body. That is to eliminate oedema and reduce or normalise the venous pressure. Such an approach can be applied clinically by careful examination and measurement of body weight. A common problem in using diuretics in this way is that renal function declines and medical treatment becomes a balance between over diuresis leading to a decline of renal function and under diuresis leading to symptoms and the retention of sodium and water.

A major advance in recent years has been realisation of the benefit of mixing diuretics [3, 11]. Thus it is perfectly reasonable for a patient to be taking a thiazide diuretic, a potassium sparing diuretic and to control and manipulate a loop diuretic with occasional use of stronger diuretics acting on the proximal tubule such as metolozone. The patient might therefore be

Table 6. Possible drugs in the treatment of chronic heart failure

Anticoagulants		
Miscellaneous	AT II inhibitors	Endothelin antagonists
	Calcium antagonists	Endopeptidase inhibitors
	Antiarrhythmics	Vasopressin inhibitors
	Lipid lowering drugs	Aminophylline
	Aspirin	Beta-2 agonists
Anabolic stimulants	Growth hormone, L-thyroxine	
Catabolic inhibitors		
Cytokine inhibitors	TNFα inhibitors, pentoxyfilline	
Gene therapy		

on no less than four different types of diuretics. They act synergistically. Patients can be instructed how to modify the dose of ferosemide according to their weight and that is advantageous particularly if it is done in conjunction with attendance at a nurse led heart failure clinic.

The recent RALES study [17] has shown the advantage of using spironolactone in patients with severe heart failure. That is now becoming standard practice. There are many potential mechanisms for the benefit of spironolactone. First, it merely acts as a further diuretic acting synergistically with others. Second it specifically inhibits some of the harmful properties of aldosterone such as the promotion of fibrosis in the heart. Third it increases the plasma potassium which might have a favourable effect on the electrical stability of the heart [5].

ACE inhibitors should be used in all patients with severe heart failure unless there is a contraindication. A common problem is a decline of renal function. The benefit in absolute terms is limited [24, 26]. In the SOLVD study there was a reduction of 4.5% from a mortality of 39.7% over a period of 41.4 months [24].

The use of positive inotropic drugs has been controversial. Table 7 contains a list of studies with such drugs where there has been no benefit or an increased mortality. The largest study ever undertaken, namely that with digoxin [8], did not show any benefit whatsoever in terms of mortality overall or in any sub-group of patients. The use of positive inotropic drugs in the long term is damaging to the heart and such drugs should not be used except to reverse an acute situation in the Intensive Care Unit. Digoxin is used in patients with atrial fibrillation and can be used if there is no other possible treatment but without the expectation of substantial benefit and none in terms of mortality.

Beta blockers have recently been shown in a number of studies (US carvedilol programme [15], CIBIS II [4], MERIT [13], BEST) and in recent metaanalyses [2, 12] to be advantageous in heart failure, possibly because of their benefit for that sub-group with coronary heart disease. They are however at the moment not proven to be of benefit in patients with NYHA

Table 7. Recent failed trials with positive inotropic drugs

Author/ Study	Date	Drug	No. of pat.	Duration (m)	Mortality
DiBianco	1989	Milrinone	230	3	8/59 Mil, 3/49 Plac, p < 0.06
Uretsky	1990	Enoximone	102	4	5 drug, 0 placebo
Xamoterol	1990	Xamoterol	516	4.25	9.1% versus 3.7%, p < 0.02
PROMISE	1991	Milrinone	1088	6.1	28% increase, p < 0.04
Narahara	1991	Enoximone	164	4	NS but adverse events
Kubo	1992	Pimobendan	198	3	5% Pim versus 6% Plac, NS
Feldman	1993	Vesnarinone	> 500	6	120 mg, increase, p < 0.01 60 mg, 62% decrease, p < 0.01
Packer	1993	Flosequinan	193	4	7/93 Flos versus 2/100 Plac
PROFILE	1994	Flosequinan	2345	12+	Increase, 21% to 46% p.< 0.002
PICO	1996	Pimobendan	331	11	Possibly increased mortality
PRIME II	1997	Ibopamine	1906	12–	Increase 25% v. 20% p < 0.02
DIG	1997	Digoxin	6800	37	No difference 35% mortality
VEST	1998	Vesnarinone	3833	10	Increase 18.9% v. 22.9% p < 0.02

Table 8. Hormonal mediators in heart failure

Constrictors	Dilators	Growth factors
Noradrenaline	ANP	Insulin
Renin/angiotensin II	Prostaglandin E2	TNF alpha
Vasopressin	& metabolites	Growth hormone
NPY	EDRF	Angiotensin II
Endothelin	Dopamine	Catecholamines
	CGRP	NO
		Cytokines
		Oxygen radicals

class IV and the most recent study which contained the sickest patients, namely the BEST study, did not show any advantage and indeed raised the possibility of harm. Beta-blockers have been until recently contraindicated in heart failure because they can cause heart failure. Much of the advantage in heart failure may be due to a benefit in those patients with coronary heart disease [18]. Further trials are currently underway in severe heart failure.

Many drugs are under investigation (Table 5). Most of these inhibit or promote one of the many metabolic pathways activated in heart failure (Table 8). These include inhibitors of TNFα, promoters of myocardial growth, inhibitors of endothelin and inhibitors of apoptosis. The causes of cachexia are being established and may lead to novel treatments [1, 14].

■ Ethical considerations

The management of patients with severe heart failure raises ethical issues which have been known for sometime but which have not been faced by the clinician in a direct manner. The mode of death in severe heart failure is often extraordinarily unpleasant being accompanied by severe cachexia, tiredness and increasing shortness of breath. Sudden death might be viewed by some as a more desirable outcome but sudden death is more common in mild heart failure than in severe heart failure. Some drugs, notably flosequinan, have been shown to improve symptoms in severe heart failure. At the same time these drugs reduce the duration of life possibly by promoting arrhythmias or by increasing the rate of loss of functional myocytes. There is then a trade off between an improved quality of life and duration of life. Under the present legal system the decision as to whether such drugs can be used is largely under the control of drug agencies. Flosequinan was taken off the market and is not available to clinicians. There is a case that clinicians, patients, healthcare groups and the public have a right to be more involved in these extremely complex human issues.

■ Non-surgical approaches

There have in the last few years been an increasing number of reports in which high technology has been used to reduce sodium retention or to prevent arrhythmias (Table 4). The use of dialysis in any form in patients with severe heart failure may have a place in the management of severe heart failure with intractable sodium retention but the exact role and the benefit of such procedures is unknown. The overall benefit is likely to be small.

A more complex matter is the issue of whether intracardiac defibrillators (ICDs) should be used in severe heart failure and in which patients. Most patients with severe heart failure do have numerous ventricular ectopics and often runs of ventricular tachycardia over a 24 h period. The number of patients dying from arrhythmias is probably lower in patients with severe heart failure than in those with mild heart failure. The benefit of ICDs might be greater in a selected population with mild heart failure than in a larger proportion of those with severe heart failure. The matter is not resolved and currently there are large trials evaluating the role of an ICD in patients with a low ejection fraction and what might be classified as severe heart failure.

■ Surgery – valves and arteries

Surgery has a major role to play in the management of severe heart failure (Table 4) and particularly when heart failure is associated with valve disorders. Examples are mitral regurgitation and aortic valve disease. A more difficult question relates to the value of coronary artery bypass surgery and those who have a dilated left ventricle, severe heart failure and severe coronary artery disease. This is a condition which is likely to lead to so-called "hibernation" of the myocardium [9, 10, 22] either due to persistent ischaemia or the result of stuttering ischaemia [25] or repeated stunning. There is strong anecdotal evidence of very substantial improvement in selected patients. Two major difficulties arise in this context. The first is how to identify and diagnose those patients most likely to benefit. Stress echocardiography, PET scanning and magnetic resonance imaging have been used for this purpose. The surgery under these circumstances does carry substantial mortality being up to 10%. The second major problem with this condition is the lack of proper evidence from controlled trials. In recent trials of new drugs the number of patients is about 3000. For a surgical trial the number would be much less because the benefit would need to be high to justify the expenditure. If the outcome event occurred in 60% of patients and this were reduced by one third to 40%, then the number of patients for an 80% power and P value of 0.05 would be less than 200. The failure to have undertaken a clinical trial is, in the view of this writer, a criticism of the cardiological community, both physicians and surgeons. There is no reason why such a surgical procedure should not be subjected to the same evaluative methods as those used for drugs. A judgement then has to be made within health systems as to whether cost justifies benefit. In this particular case the benefit would have to be substantial to justify the cost and under those circumstances the number of patients required in a randomised trial is reasonably small and such a study could clearly be undertaken.

■ Surgery – transplantation

Transplantation is discussed elsewhere in this Symposium. The subject is, however, relevant to the management of severe heart failure because of the need to judge when medical approaches should be abandoned and the patient put forward for transplantation. There are many difficult issues in this area. Many patients being put forward for heart transplantation come into the hospital in NYHA IV with severe heart failure. Often these patients do respond reasonably well to sophisticated medical treatment and are then in class NYHA II or III despite having been referred for transplantation. The result is that in some studies the management of these patients under medical treatment appears to be almost as good as transplantation [25]. The long-term follow-up of patients treated medically may show that the exercise capacity of these patients is rather similar to those who have undergone transplantation. The point which emerges is that it is important that patients being considered for transplantation are either in a stable condition with severe heart failure or are deteriorating in such a way that reversal of that deterioration is most improbable.

The management of patients after transplantation has improved greatly in the last two decades. As a consequence the outcome has improved. The more careful selection of patients is another factor which has contributed to improvement in outcome. However there is a weakness in that argument because selection of patients with a more favourable outcome after transplantation tends to select out those patients who are less ill. Thus often patients are now not considered for transplantation if there are severe renal abnormalities (even if due to pre-renal failure) or abnormalities of hepatic function. Some of the overall improvement in outcome may therefore be merely the consequence of undertaking transplantation on a more healthy population. If that is so then the decision to refer a patient for transplantation becomes considerably more complex. In very severe heart failure the prognosis is so poor that it is obvious that transplantation has a benefit and a trial is not required. If more healthy patients are selected the issue is less clear and there would be a need for a clinical trial of transplantation against medical treatment. That is a proposal which has never been considered previously. Some may argue that such a trial is impossible and certainly in some groups of patients that would be true. For example it would be difficult to argue for such a trial in very young patients with dilated cardiomyopathy with established severe and progressive heart failure.

■ Surgery – devices and surgery for remodelling

In the last few decades there has been an attempt to manufacture an artificial heart. Failure of this enterprise was followed by realisation that the major problem in patients with heart failure was left ventricular heart failure. As a consequence numerous mechanical devices, known as left ventricular assist devices, (Heartmate, Thoratec, Novacor) have come onto the market. These are devices are large, present considerable difficulties with regard to surgical implantation and are prone to infection and thrombosis. Newer devices are currently being evaluated which are small axial flow pumps. These have the advantage that the surgical procedure is more simple and, in theory at least, these devices could be removed from the heart if there were to be recovery of myocardial function. Rather than repeat what has happened in the past these devices should be introduced into medical practice in formal programmes which will demonstrate benefit or otherwise. The arguments against such a protocol driven procedure and the resistance to evaluating such devices in a methodical manner are rather similar to views expressed several decades ago about placebo groups in trials of drugs with heart failure.

■ Future

The future over the next fifteen years in the management of patients with severe heart failure will be a race between the development of mechanical devices and advances in biology (Table 9). I would anticipate that successful mechanical devices will become available and will be used extensively in patients with severe heart failure. At the same time there is going to be an explosion of activity with regard to the biology of heart failure. This will focus on the mechanisms concerned with promoting growth of myocytes and preventing loss of myocytes in the heart. Inhibitors of apoptosis will be tested. Gene therapy will be devised to activate growth in the heart. Myocytes will be grown from more primitive cell types, be they stem cells, fibroblasts, bone marrow cells or skeletal muscle cells. As many as 20% of myocytes in the human heart have two nuclei and these cells could divide by a process other than mitosis. It is heresy to believe that mitosis can occur in the myocardium but it is possible that mechanisms will be found for overcoming the inhibitors of mitosis or that primitive cells will be found in the myocardium which can develop into cardiac myocytes. New myocardial tissue will require a blood supply. Developments in gene therapy for promoting arteriogenesis and angiogenesis will occur at the same time as advances in promoting myocyte growth. Heart failure is a disease for which new therapeutic strategies must be found (Table 10) in order to

Table 9. Molecular biology – probable advances

- Proliferation of remaining myocytes and migration to infarct area
- Induction of angiogenesis to support new myocytes
- Cell transplantation
- Conversion of fibroblasts or skeletal muscle cells to cardiac muscle cells in ischaemic area
- Cell growth of myocytes from embryonic cells, marrow cells or stem cells
- Division and growth of adult mammalian cardiac myocytes
- Vaccines for infection and inflammation in arteries
- Pharmacological control of smooth muscle cell

Table 10. Future directions in the treatment of heart failure

Current position
- Mortality, symptoms, hospitalisation, exercise capacity, events benefitted
- Haemodynamics restored towards normal, heart size reduced
- Regression of hypertrophy, myocardial biology improved

But mortality and morbidity remain high – new concepts
- Nature of control of extracellular structure – ? site of memory
- Cell transplantation
- Control of cell division (mitotic division or hyperplasia)
- Control of cell growth, modify apoptosis, promote angiogenesis

overcome the inevitable consequence of the loss of functioning myocytes. At present we tinker with the response of the body to dysfunction of the heart as a pump and are pleased to reduce symptoms and prolong life to a small degree; for the future we must have greater ambitions to resolve the problem by replacing the lost myocardium.

■ References

1. Anker SD, Ponikowski PP, Clark AL et al (1999) Cytokines and neurohormones relating to body composition alterations in the wasting syndrome of chronic heart failure. Eur Heart J 20:683–693
2. Avezum A, Tsuyuki RT, Pogue J, Yusuf S (1998) Beta-blocker therapy for congestive heart failure: a systemic overview and critical appraisal of the published trials. Can J Cardiol 14:1045–1053
3. Channer KS, McLean KA, Lawson-Mathew P, Richardson M (1994) Combination therapy in severe heart failure: a randomised controlled trial. Br Heart J 71:146–150
4. CIBIS-II Investigators and Committees (1999) The Cardiac Insufficiency Bisoprolol Study II (CIBIS-II): a randomised trial. Lancet 353:9–13
5. Cooper HA, Dries DL, Davis CE, Shen YL, Domanski MJ (1999) Diuretics and risk of arrhythmic death in patients with left ventricular dysfunction. Circulation 100:1311–1315
6. Cowie MR, Mosterd A, Wood DA et al (1997) The epidemiology of heart failure. Eur Heart J 18:208–225.
7. The Criteria Committee of the New York Heart Association (1994) 1994 revisions to classification of functional capacity and objective assessment of patients with diseases of the heart. Circulation 90:644–645
8. The Digitalis Investigation Group (1997) The effect of digoxin on mortality and morbidity in patients with heart failure. N Engl J Med 336:525–533
9. Ferrari R, La Canna G, Giubbini R et al (1994) Left ventricular dysfunction due to stunning and hibernation in patients. Cardiovasc Drugs Ther 8:371–380
10. Kannel WB, Cupples A (1988) Epidemiology and risk profile of cardiac failure. Cardiovasc Drugs Ther 2:387–395
11. Kiyingi A, Field MJ, Pawsey CC, Yiannikas J, Lawrence JR, Arter WJ (1990) Metolazone in treatment of severe refractory congestive cardiac failure. Lancet 335:29–31
12. Lechat P, Packer M, Chalon S, Cucherat M, Arab T, Boissel JP (1998) Clinical effects of beta-adrenergic blockade in chronic heart failure: a meta-analysis of double-blind, placebo-controlled, randomized trials. Circulation 98:1184–1191
13. MERIT-HF Study Group (1999) Effect of metoprolol CR/XL in chronic heart failure: Metoprolol CR/XL Randomised Intervention Trial in Congestive Heart Failure (MERIT-HF). Lancet 353:2001–2007
14. Niebauer J, Volk HD, Kemp M et al (1999) Endotoxin and immune activation in chronic heart failure: a prospective cohort study. Lancet 353:1838–1842
15. Packer M, Bristow MR, Cohn JN et al (1996) The effect of carvedilol on morbidity and mortality in patients with chronic heart failure. N Engl J Med 334:1349–1355
16. Parameshwar J, Keegan J, Sparrow J, Sutton GC, Poole-Wilson PA (1992) Predictors of prognosis in severe heart failure. Am Heart J 123:421–426
17. Pitt B, Zannad F, Remme WJ et al (1999) The effect of spironolactone on morbidity and mortality in patients with severe heart failure. N Engl J Med 341:709–717

18. Poole-Wilson PA (1999) The Cardiac Insufficiency Bisoprolol Study II. Lancet 353:1360
19. Poole-Wilson PA (1996) The clinical causes of heart failure. In: Dargie HJ, McMurray JJV, Poole-Wilson PA (eds) Managing Heart Failure in Primary Care. 1 ed. Blackwell Healthcare Communications, London, pp 11–22
20. Poole-Wilson PA (1997) History, definition and classification of heart failure. In: Poole-Wilson PA, Colucci WS, Massie BM, Chatterjee K, Coats AJS (eds) Heart Failure. 1 ed. Churcill Livingstone, New York, pp 269–277
21. Purcell IF, Poole-Wilson PA (1999) Heart failure: why and how to define it? Eur J Heart Failure 1:7–10
22. Rahimtoola SH, Griffith GC (1989) The hibernating myocardium. Am Heart J 117:211–221
23. Sapin PM, Koch G, Blauwet MB, McCarthy JJ, Hinds SW, Gettes LS (1991) Identification of false positive exercise tests with use of electrocardiographic criteria: a possible role for atrial repolarisation waves. J Am Coll Cardiol 18:127–135
24. The SOLVD Investigators (1991) Effect of enalapril on survival in patients with reduced left ventricular ejection fractions and congestive heart failure. N Engl J Med 325:293–302
25. Stevenson LJ, Sietsema K, Tillisch JH et al (1990) Execise capacity for survivors of cardiac transplantation or sustained medical therapy for stable heart failure. Circulation 81:78–85
26. Swedberg K, Kjekshus J, Snapinn S (1999) Long-term survival in severe heart failure in patients treated with enalapril. Ten year follow-up of CONSENSUS. Eur Heart J20:136–139

Author's address:

Prof. Dr. P. A. Poole-Wilson, MD FRCP FACC FESC
Cardiac Medicine, National Heart & Lung Institute,
Imperial College School of Medicine, National Heart & Lung Institute
Dovehouse Street, London SW3 6LY, UK
E-mail: p.poole-wilson@ic.ac.uk

CHAPTER **3** **Heart transplantation for cardiomyopathy – therapeutic gold standard?**

W. Harringer, M. Wirsing, H.-W. Künsebeck,
K. Pethig, and A. Haverich

▦ Introduction

The number of heart transplantations steadily increased worldwide during the 1980s and has plateaued since 1990 around 3500–4000 annually performed procedures. Meanwhile, more than 48 000 such interventions have been reported during the last 20 years [7]. Improved immunosuppression, antibiotic, and antimycotic therapies have led to better survival and long-term results even in patients with multiple concomitant diseases. Thus, cardiac transplantation has evolved from an experimental procedure to the therapeutic gold standard for patients with end-stage heart failure, refractory to medical treatment. Limitations of this procedure are evident with lack of available donor organs, side effects of immunosuppression (e.g., hypertension, renal insufficiency, osteoporosis) as well as an increased malignancy rate and chronic allograft rejection being the most predominant. Alternatively, new organ preserving surgical strategies as well as mechanical cardiac support devices have evolved, aiming at improvements in patient symptoms and quality of life as well as survival. Evaluation of all these techniques has to be balanced carefully against the results achieved with heart transplantation during the last two decades. The aim of this article is to present our management combined with long-term results in this patient group.

▦ Indications and recipient selection

Limited availability of donor organs, the cost of the procedure, and intensive follow-up care requires careful recipient evaluation and selection. Criteria have evolved over time, are continuously refined, and might differ slightly from center to center based on experience, priorities, and attitudes. They can provide a guideline for recipient selection, but the decision for patient acceptance as a transplant candidate has to be made on an individual basis involving all members of the transplant team.

Most centers accept patients up to 60 years for heart transplantation and as in other solid organ transplant candidates there is no lower age limit, albeit the number of transplants in children, especially infants is low. Adequate compliance with medical therapy and absence of alcohol or drug abuse remains mandatory for all transplant candidates.

Current indications for cardiac transplantation includes patients with end-stage heart failure (NYHA III–IV) and an estimated 1-year survival <50%. Left ventricular ejection fraction should be <20% with a cardiac index <2 l/min/m^3 and elevated left ventricular filling pressures. More recently, reduced maximum oxygen consumption (<14 ml/kg/min) has been identified as a very reliable predictor for poor prognosis in heart failure [8]. Priority should be given to patients with malignant ventricular arrhythmia, active ischemia, right ventricular failure, and hyponatremia.

Extracardiac malignancies, elevated pulmonary arteriolar resistance (>6 Wood units or >480 dyn×s×cm^{-5}) despite intensive combined therapy with vasodilator and inotropic agents for several days, irreversible renal or hepatic dysfunction as well as severe pulmonary disease (FEV1 <1.5 l/s) are absolute contraindications for heart transplantation. Relative contraindications include acute concomitant diseases (infection, pulmonary emboli, peptic ulcer, cerebral ischemia) as well as diabetes including significant secondary organ damage.

■ Immunosuppression and surveillance

Today, most centers use a triple-drug immunosuppressive regimen (cyclosporine A, prednisolone, azathioprine) following thoracic organ transplantation. Additionally, induction therapy is applied with poly- or monoclonal antibodies (e.g., ATG, OKT3) and pulsed steroids starting immediately postoperative. Intravenous cyclosporine A is usually administered within 6 hours postoperatively. The initial dose (1 mg/kg) is switched to an oral preparation and increased within the following 1 to 2 weeks up to 5–10 mg/kg depending on renal and hepatic function. Cyclosporine A serum levels (monoclonal assay) should range between 250±50 ng/ml for the first year with reduction to 150±50 ng/ml for the following years. Patients also receive 1–2 mg/kg azathioprine with a target white blood cell count of 4000 cells/mm^3 or greater. Prednisolone (1000 mg i.v.) is administered intraoperatively followed by 3 doses of 125 mg (heart) or 250 mg (lung and heart-lung) at 12-hour-intervals. Prednisolone maintenance therapy is started on the second postoperative day (initially 0.5 mg/kg and tapered to 0.1 mg/kg within 1 year). More recently, tacrolimus and mycofenolic acid have gained increased acceptance in routine immunosuppression following heart transplantation. Additional drugs, currently under clinical or experimental investigation, will influence patient management significantly in the coming years. The aim of the new pharmaceutical developments is more specific and less toxic immunosuppression with a greater impact on prevention of allograft vasculopathy.

Cardiac rejection is predominantly diagnosed by transvenous endomyocardial biopsies. Non-invasive diagnosis of myocardial function with echocardiography, however, gains increased importance, especially beyond the first postoperative year. In our center, standard monitoring of patients presenting an uncomplicated course after 1 year is done by echocardiography alone with transvenous biopsies being performed only during routine coronary angiography once a year.

Severe rejection episodes including myocyte necrosis are treated with pulsed steroids (prednisolone 500 mg/day for 3 days) with rebiopsy 7 days after completion of rejection therapy. Steroid resistant rejection or rejection with hemodynamic compromise are treated more aggressively, using monoclonal or polyclonal antibodies.

▪ Outcome

International

The number of heart transplantations has plateaued since 1990 at around 3800–4000 procedures per year as recorded in the International Society for Heart and Lung Transplantation database. Overall, international 1-year-survival rate is 79% with a following constant mortality rate of 4% per year [7]. Interestingly, no significant survival improvement has occurred when comparing patients transplanted between 1986–90 and patients transplanted between 1991–95. Increasing donor and recipient age as well as expanding indications during these time intervals might have had some influence on survival statistics.

Hannover

Starting with heart transplantations in July 1983, a continuously growing thoracic organ transplantation program has been developed at Hannover Medical School with a total of 650 heart transplantations performed in 617 patients. Indications for transplantation were dilated cardiomyopathy in 58%, coronary artery disease in 31%, and 6% others; 5% of these patients underwent redotransplantation. Retransplant patients were initially included in survival data analysis from the time of their primary transplant.

Comparing the transplant indications from 1983 to 1989 (n = 316) and 1990 to 11/1999 (n = 334) there was an increasing rate in patients with coronary artery disease from 30% to 33% and a decreasing rate in patients with dilated cardiomyopathy from 60% to 55% (Fig. 1).

Although a small but significant improvement in survival could be shown between these time intervals, little is known about graft function, quality of live, and overall success after long-term follow-up (≥10 years after heart transplantation).

We therefore evaluated in detail the outcome of 120 patients (98 male, 22 female) who had undergone heart transplantation at Hannover Medical

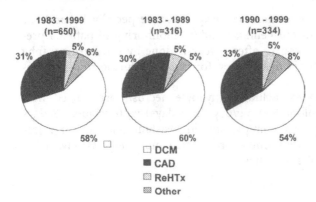

Fig. 1. Indications for heart transplantation at Hannover Medical School (7/1983–11/1999); *DCM* dilative cardiomyopathy, *CAD* ischemic cardiomyopathy, *ReHTx* retransplantation)

School from 1983 to 1989, resulting in a mean follow-up of 11±0.7 years [4]. Mean age of the recipients at the time of transplantation was 42 years; mean donor age was 26 years, with 83 male (69.2%) and 27 female donors (22.5%) (10 with missing data). The indication for heart transplantation and cause of heart failure in these 120 patients was dilated cardiomyopathy in 69 patients (58%), coronary artery disease in 42 patients (35%), and other diseases (valve related, endocardial fibrosis, and hypertrophic cardiomyopathy) in 9 patients (7%).

Immunosuppression and close monitoring of all patients was performed by our transplant service according to the protocol described above. Patients with compromised renal function (creatinine levels >150 mmol/l) were treated with adapted cyclosporine levels depending on the individual course. Standard drugs were used for the treatment of hypercholesterolemia and hypertension. The frequency of examination in our outpatient department was at least every three months beyond the first year after transplantation.

Echocardiographic measurements were performed using a Hewlett-Packard 2500 ultrasound imaging system with a 2.5- or 5.0-MHz transducer from standard windows. Left ventricular diastolic and systolic dimensions and fractional shortening were measured using standard M-mode techniques. Left ventricular mass (LVM) was calculated from M-mode measurements of left ventricular enddiastolic diameter, interventricular septum thickness, and left ventricular posterior wall thickness, using the formula modified by Devereux and Reichek [3].

Quality of life assessment of surviving patients together with psychological, social, and occupational status was evaluated by standardized questionnaires and interviews by a specialized psychiatrist.

▨ Survival

Overall actuarial survival rate at the present time is 81% at 1 year, 70% at 5 years, and 51% at 10 years. A tendency for improved survival could be observed in patients with dilated cardiomyopathy during long-term follow-up when compared to patients with coronary artery disease (10 yr.: 52% vs. 38%), but the difference did not reach statistical significance (n.s., log-rank test) (Fig. 2).

▨ Long-term morbidity and mortality

During the follow-up period, 62 patients died and 58 (48%) are presently alive and were available for further detailed analysis. The most common underlying cause for death in these 62 patients was chronic graft failure due to CAVD (cardiac allograft vascular disease) in 39%, demonstrating that CAVD remains the main complication impairing long-term survival. Endothelial dysfunction and multifocal myo-intimal hyperplasia, modified by vascular remodeling processes, represent the pathophysiological basis of this accelerated coronary syndrome. Additional causes of death were attributed to right heart failure in 18%, infections in 11%, and malignancies in 11% (Fig. 3). The main reason for death during the first year was acute graft rejection in 40% of the patients.

The new development of malignant tumors is one of the major side effects of chronic immunosuppression. The current estimate of the risk of malignancy after heart transplantation is about 3–5%/year [9]. Among our long-term patients, malignancy was the cause of death in 11%. Additionally, neoplasm appeared in the long-term survivors as well (n = 8, 14%): three patients developed lymphoma, two patients lung cancer, one patient colon cancer, and one hematological neoplasia. Currently, all of these patients are still alive after successful surgical or medical treatment. Overall, about 25% of our transplanted patients suffered from malignant neoplasm

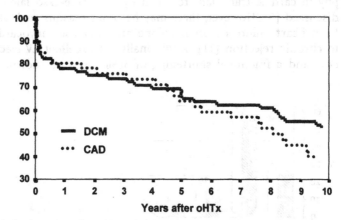

Fig. 2. Actuarial survival after heart transplantation at the Hannover Medical School (n = 650); *DCM* dilative cardiomyopathy, *CAD* ischemic cardiomyopathy

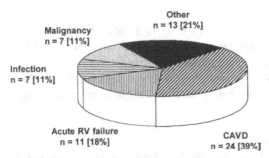

Fig. 3. Causes of death 10 years after heart transplantation (n=62)

during the 10 year period. This demonstrates the magnitude of the problem and represents a major challenge for future improvements in immunosuppressive strategies [2].

▨ Graft function

Exercise tolerance in long-term survivors proved to be excellent (Fig. 4). The most recent coronary angiography in our survivors showed no signs of graft vasculopathy in 27 patients (46%), 15 had a luminal obstruction of grade 1 or 2, and only 16 patients had high grade vasculopathy (grade 3 or 4) [10].

Cardiac allograft function was additionally assessed until now in 42 of the 58 patients by color Doppler echocardiography. The mean observation period was 12 years postoperatively. Left ventricular dimensions were predominantly within the normal range (LVEDD 46 mm). The left and right atrium showed normal dimensions as well (38 and 42 mm). Calculating left ventricular mass revealed left ventricular hypertrophy as a frequent finding with a mean LV_{mass} of 251.8 g (Normal range: 177 g±40 for male and 127 g±30 for female patients) [12]. As the main reason for hypertrophy in cardiac transplant recipient cyclosporine-associated hypertension is discussed [5]. However, there may be other reasons such as fluid retention from heart failure or prednisolone and increased myocardial fibrosis due to chronic rejection [11]. Additionally, an excellent LV ejection fraction of 64% and a fractional shortening of 35% could be shown. In contrast, left

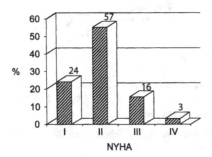

Fig. 4. NYHA – classification of patients 10 years after heart transplantation (n=58)

Table 1. Functional parameters of cardiac allograft more than 10 years after orthotopic heart transplantation

N	Years post HTX	EF (%)	FS (%)	LVEDD (mm)	LVESD (mm)	RVEDD (mm)	TI > II (N)	TKR (N)
42	12±5	63±6	35±9	46±5	29±5	37±9	29	3

atrial function was significantly impaired following the standard transplantation technique with an atrial filling wave detectable in only 21 of 42 patients (50%).

Right ventricular analysis demonstrated an increased diameter in the majority of our patients with tricuspid valve insufficiency being present in 69% (Table 1). Enlargement of the right ventricle and incompetence of the tricuspid valve is seen in most cases already 24 hours after the operation. These alterations are related to long periods of global myocardial ischemia and elevated pulmonary resistance. Tricuspid insufficiency can be aggravated during follow-up by damage to the subvalvular apparatus as a result of myocardial biopsies leading to chordal rupture [5].

▪ Quality of life

Quality of live is a discrete but increasingly important parameter to assess treatment strategies beyond survival and organ function. It is related to determinants like physical and psychological integrity, function in every day life, and social integration. In our study 47 patients more than 10 years after heart transplantation took part in a psychological follow-up performed with standardized questionnaires and interviews. The most frequent complaints were back pain (34%), dermatological problems (15%), and exhaustion (19%) with a slight increase between one and 10 years after cardiac transplantation. More than one third of our patients complained about a lack of concentration as well as impotence, whereas change of appearance worried only 15%, compared to 38% within the first year of transplantation.

Despite these complaints, contentment with the way of life after transplantation was rated very high. Overall satisfaction with the financial situation could be documented in 65% and with family life in more than 90% of the patients. Significant improvement of physical functions with an increased satisfaction were seen in 72% of patients after transplantation compared to 9% before transplantation (Fig. 5 a, b). In contrast to other publications about long-term follow-up after heart transplantation, depression was not a major problem in our patient cohort [11]. Of the patients on the waiting list, 40% complained about depression, one year after transplantation 15%, and after ten years 17%.

Finally, for the vast majority of our long-term survivors expectations in cardiac transplantation were completely fulfilled. More importantly, 80% of

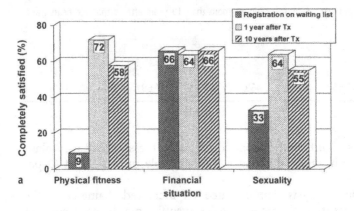

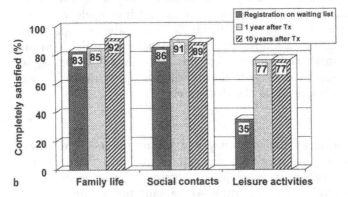

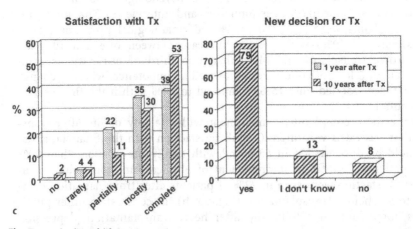

Fig. 5a–c. Quality of life 10 years after heart transplantation. Overall satisfaction and acceptance of procedure

Table 2. Selected predictors of long-term survival after heart transplantation

	All patients (n = 120)	Long-term survivors (n = 58)	Deceased patients (n = 62)	P Value
Recipient age (yrs)	42 ± 12	42 ± 12	42 ± 12	0.8
Donor age (yrs)	26 ± 9	24 ± 9	27 ± 8	0.08
Ischemic time (min)	138 ± 43	137 ± 43	138 ± 43	0.9
HLA mismatch	4.6 ± 0.9	4.6 ± 1.0	4.6 ± 0.9	0.8
ATG treatment	99	46	53	0.7
Number of antihypertensive drugs at year 1		1.2 ± 0.9	1.0 ± 0.9	0.7

them would accept a heart transplantation as a therapeutic option once again (Fig. 5 c).

▪ Analysis of predictive factors

Analysis of predictive factors for survival was performed comparing characteristics of long-term survivors with deceased patients. The following variables were analyzed: recipient age, donor age, sex, cytomegalovirus status, HLA mismatch, ischemic time, ATG induction treatment, immunosuppression (mean dose/day of cyclosporine A, prednisolone and azathioprine) as well as lipid levels and the number of antihypertensive drugs at one year post-transplant. Using a univariate and a multivariate logistic regression analysis, no independent predictors of long-term survival for more than 10 years could be identified. A selection of variables between groups is presented in Table 2.

▪ Conclusion

Long-term survival, allograft function and quality of life in patients undergoing cardiac transplantation is excellent compared to an otherwise deleterious natural course of the disease. As our patients demonstrate, nearly 50% will survive a 10-year-period with acceptable exercise tolerance and quality of life. Thus, this therapeutic strategy clearly has evolved from an experimental approach to the gold standard in the management of patients with heart failure, refractory to medical management. However, major obstacles remain and require further improvements in the management of such patients. First of all, limitation of a more widespread use is a clear shortage of donor organs despite a significant increase in donor age during the last decade. Additionally, chronic allograft vasculopathy and development of malignancies represent a constant threat to the postoperative course of these patients. Intensified research and modification of immunosuppressive strategies as well as tolerance induction protocols might lead to further risk reduction with even better outcome of patients after heart transplantation.

▪ References

1. Bhatia SJS, Kirshenbaum JM, Shemin RJ, Cohn LH, Collins JJ, Di Sesa VJ, Young PJ, Mudge GH, Sutton MGSJ (1987) Time course of resolution of pulmonary hypertension and right ventricular remodelling after orthotopic cardiac transplantation. Circulation 76:819–826
2. Constanzo-Nordin MR, Cooper DK, Jessup M, Renlund DG, Robinson JA, Rose EA (1993) Task Force 6: future developments. J Am Coll Cardiol 22:1–64
3. Devereux RB, Reichek N (1977) Echocardiographic determination of left ventricular mass in man. Anatomic validation of the method. Circulation 1977, 55:613–18
4. Fraund S, Pethig K, Franke U, Wahlers T, Harringer W, Cremer J, Fieguth HG, Oppelt P, Haverich A (1999) Ten-year-survival after heart transplantation: palliative procedure or successful long term treatment? Heart 82:47–51
5. Gill EA, Borrego C, Bray B, Renlund DG, Hammond E, Gilbert EM (1995) Left ventricular mass increases during cardiac allograft vascular rejection. J Am Coll Cardiol 25:922–926
6. Hetzer R, Albert W, Hummel M, Pasic M, Loebe M, Warnecke H, Haverich A, Borst HG (1997) Status of patients presently living 9 to 13 years after orthotopic heart transplantation. Ann Thorac Surg 64:1661–1668
7. Hosenpud JD, Bennett LE, Keck BM, Fiol B, Boucek MM, Novick RJ (1999) The Registry of the International Society for Heart and Lung Transplantation: sixteenth official report – 1999. J Heart Lung Transplant 18:611–626
8. Mancini DM, Eisen H, Kussmaul W, Mull R, Edmunds LH Jr, Wilson JR (1991) Value of peak exercise oxygen consumption for optimal timing of cardiac transplantation in ambulatory patients with heart failure. Circulation 83:778–786
9. Miller LW, Schlant R, Kobashigawa J, Spencer K, Renlund DG (1993) Task Force 5: Complications. J Am Coll Cardiol 22:1–64
10. Pethig K, Besser K, Heublein B, Wahlers T, Harringer W, Haverich A (1999) Coronary vasculopathy after heart transplantation – effect of temporal onset, severity and progression on long-term prognosis. Z Kardiol 88:498–506
11. Robbins R, Barlow C, Oyer P, Hunt SA, Miller L, Reitz BA, Stinson E, Shumway E (1999) Thirty years of cardiac transplantation at Stanford University. J Thorac Cardiovasc Surg 117:939–951
12. Schirmer H, Linde P, Rasmussen K (1999) Prevalence of left ventricular hypertrophy in a general population. Eur Heart J 6:429–436

Author's address:

Dr. W. Harringer
Division of Thoracic and Cardiovascular Surgery
Hannover Medical School
30623 Hannover, Germany
E-mail: harringer@thg.mh-hannover.de

CHAPTER **4** **Cardiac assistance from skeletal muscle: achieving a viable and appropriately transformed graft**

S. SALMONS

■ Summary

For some years the surgical treatment of end-stage cardiac failure has been restricted to cardiac transplantation. The discovery that adult mammalian skeletal muscle is capable of undergoing adaptive change, through which it can acquire a markedly increased resistance to fatigue, has revived interest in the possibility of diverting a skeletal muscle from its normal function to perform in a cardiac assist role. For procedures based on this approach to be successful, the skeletal muscle graft must remain viable and acquire a functional profile appropriate to the task. Recent work shows that we have a better chance of achieving these objectives if we re-examine both the working conditions and the way in which we prepare the skeletal muscle graft to meet them.

■ Introduction

Background

End-stage heart failure is a common, debilitating, and ultimately fatal condition for which there is still no adequate solution. For some years heart transplantation has been the only available surgical remedy. It can be offered only to selected patients, and its benefits have to be weighed against the high cost of surgery and the costs and unwanted side-effects of lifelong immunosuppression. The number of heart failure patients that can be treated by transplants is severely limited by a shortage of donors. As a result, many patients are excluded from transplant lists by reason of age or complicating illness, and 20–30% die while awaiting a transplant. The availability of xenografts from transgenic pigs or baboons could reduce the waiting list mortality but would carry the additional risk of infection by latent animal viruses [23], and it does nothing to address the other problems. Ventricular reduction surgery has attracted interest, but in most centres to date it has carried a high peri-operative mortality. For an adequate assessment of its benefits we await the outcome of properly conducted clinical trials [29]. Mechanical artificial hearts will continue to be used mainly as a bridge-to-transplant. Even if all the problems of biocompatibility, haemocompatibility, and infection were solved, the continuous presence of an external power supply represents an unacceptable psychological challenge to the patient in the longer term [36].

Skeletal muscle assist

Against this background, a surgical approach to cardiac assist based on the use of the patient's own skeletal muscle is an attractive prospect. As an excitable tissue, skeletal muscle allows the expenditure of a small amount of energy (needed to stimulate the motor nerve) to trigger the release of a much larger amount of energy, derived ultimately from the normal intake of food and oxygen. Muscle converts that energy with great efficiency into mechanical work, so that a suitably deployed muscle can share the workload of the patient's ailing heart, offering not only relief of symptoms but also some potential for myocardial recovery. The use of endogenous tissue avoids the risks, debilitating side-effects, and costs associated with long-term immunosuppression, as well as the problem of donor availability. The costs are mainly those associated with the surgical procedure itself, including the implantable stimulator used to activate the grafted muscle.

Conditioning

The literature from the early years of this century contains several examples of the intrathoracic use of skeletal muscle as a surgical biomaterial for enlargement or repair. The notion of exploiting the contractile function of skeletal muscle to provide cardiac assistance dates from the experimental work of Kantrowitz [20]. However, these and other early experiments were thwarted by the problem of fatigue. The heart of an average person has to work at a rate of 1.3 W–3 W to pump blood around the body. Skeletal muscles can easily work at these high levels for short periods, but they quickly fatigue if required to do so without periods of rest. The problem was regarded as insuperable and, despite intermittent interest, the approach was abandoned.

In 1979, my group (then in Birmingham, England), joined forces with Dr. L.W. Stephenson's group (then in Philadelphia, U.S.A.). We had a new ingredient to inject: the discovery that, over a period of time, skeletal muscles could change their physiological, biochemical, and structural characteristics to accommodate a more demanding pattern of use [37, 41, 44, 47]. This adaptive response includes changes in metabolism and blood supply [41], and we were able to show that a muscle transformed in this way could work continuously, like the heart [2]. The broad basis for the use of skeletal muscle in cardiac assistance was thus established:

- induction of phenotypic changes that make the muscle resistant to fatigue, a process now referred to as 'conditioning';

■ a series of surgical manoevres in which a non-essential muscle is diverted from its normal role, transferred into the chest, and configured so as to assist the heart;

■ implantation of an electrical stimulator that is triggered by the electrical activity of the patient's heart and makes the muscle contract at the right moment during the cardiac cycle.

■ Main approaches to skeletal muscle assistance

Cardiomyoplasty

Until now the clinical use of skeletal muscle assistance has been confined to cardiomyoplasty and aortomyoplasty. In these procedures the latissimus dorsi muscle is wrapped around existing structures: the ventricles of the heart in cardiomyoplasty, and the ascending or descending aorta in aortomyoplasty. Experience with aortomyoplasty is limited as yet, in terms of the number of patients (currently about 20 worldwide) and the duration of follow-up. Cardiomyoplasty has been carried out in over 1500 patients worldwide and there is now a substantial body of follow-up data [9, 14, 30, 57, 60]. Although there is still some argument about the mechanism, a consensus is emerging that the main benefits derive from a girdling action of the muscle, which tends to prevent further enlargement of the ventricles and in some documented cases actually reduces their size [5, 21, 32]. Cardiomyoplasty and aortomyoplasty have the considerable advantage that they do not expose blood to new interfaces. However, they suffer from one serious limitation: the geometry of the wrap is dictated by the size and shape of the existing organs. In some ways the consequences of this limitation are obvious: in cardiomyoplasty, a grossly hypertrophied heart may be too large to be covered effectively by the patient's latissimus dorsi muscle, and in aortomyoplasty the small lumen of the aorta restricts the stroke volume which can be achieved by compressing it. But just as important as these anatomical considerations are the loading conditions which the fixed geometry imposes on the muscle wrap, since they constrain the muscle to operate far from the peak of its power curve [42, 43].

Skeletal muscle ventricles

The power available for assisting the heart can be harnessed to striking effect if the grafted muscle is formed into a separate auxiliary pump, or skeletal muscle ventricle. This can then be connected to the circulation to provide synchronous or counterpulsatory assistance [1, 3, 34, 58]. In this approach the only constraints are the size, shape, and fibre orientation of the latissimus dorsi (or other muscle) that is available; subject only to these limitations, factors such as cavity volume, wall thickness, and direction of wrap are all within the control of the surgeon and can, given the appropriate basic knowledge, be optimised to provide the maximum pumping performance of which the muscle is capable. Set against this functional potential is the need to ensure that the introduction of such a device into the patient's circulation does not cause thrombus formation, with the attendant risks of obstruction of flow through the device and embolism to vital organs. Careful study of the flow behaviour in model ventricles [49–52] indicates that these problems can be overcome. Indeed, in the Detroit laboratories of our collaborator, Dr. L.W. Stephenson, skeletal muscle ventricles have pumped as diastolic counterpulsators in dogs for over 2 years [59] and some have since functioned in circulation for more than 4 years (work in progress).

■ Optimising the functionality of the skeletal muscle graft

Maintaining the viability of the graft

Most patients who undergo cardiomyoplasty enjoy an improved quality of life, but between 15 and 20% do not benefit from the procedure [11]. Furthermore, in a review of 127 patients who underwent cardiomyoplasty over a 10-year period, the two-year survival rate was found to be less than 60% [14]. A high proportion of deaths are undoubtedly due to arrhythmias, but this does not explain the failure in other cases to ameliorate the clinical condition, or at least to arrest its progression. Attention has therefore focused on deterioration of the muscle wrap, of which there is evidence both from animals [4, 10, 12, 24, 35] and man [19, 31]. The crucial question is whether such damage is inevitable or whether it could be avoided by modifying existing protocols. The answer to this question is relevant not just to cardiomyoplasty but to all forms of skeletal muscle assistance.

Graft damage, involving replacement of muscle by fibrous tissue and fat, appears to be caused by a combination of factors, including changes in vascular conformation, loss of resting tension, and chronic electrical stimulation [12, 40]. Of these factors, ischaemia, particularly of the distal part of the muscle, is increasingly regarded as the most important. The ischaemia arises when the flap is lifted, because it is necessary to divide perforating branches of the intercostal arteries that enter the distal part of the muscle; sacrifice of these so-called collateral vessels has been shown to cause damage in both sheep [12] and goats [16]. Although a passive graft might survive this intervention, these grafts are far from passive; on the contrary, they are metabolically challenged by the stimulation needed to condition and to activate the muscle. The combination of an impaired blood supply with a greatly increased energy demand creates the conditions for damage [40].

Mannion and his colleagues thought that this problem could be overcome by introducing a 'vascular delay' of 3 weeks after reconfiguring the muscle and before initiating stimulation [26, 27]. The idea was that this would provide time for neovascularisation, extending the area effectively perfused by the thoracodorsal artery. The clinical cardiomyoplasty protocol that is most widely used includes such a delay, in this case of 2 weeks [15]. The problem is that it also delays the benefit that the patient might otherwise be deriving from the operation. Moreover it is not necessarily effective: even with these precautions the additive damaging effects of stimulation and division of collateral vessels can still be demonstrated [12, 16]. Better results have been obtained by implementing a true vascular delay, in which the collateral vessels are divided but the latissimus dorsi muscle is left *in situ* for 10 d before elevating it as a graft [7, 8].

Although it is impossible to avoid loss of the perforating arteries, the anatomy of the vascular supply to the latissimus dorsi muscle offers a potential solution to the problem that has been overlooked. Our recent experiments in sheep have confirmed the existence of arterial anastomoses that connect the vascular trees of the thoracodorsal artery and perforating arteries in the latissimus dorsi muscle, and we have shown that these anastomoses are functional under normal physiological conditions of pressure and flow [48]. Such anastomotic channels should enable blood delivered by the thoracodorsal artery to perfuse the distal region of the mobilised muscle through the existing arterial networks without the need to wait for neovascularisation. Why, then, does the latissimus dorsi muscle become ischaemic at all? Surgical mobilisation involves handling and cooling of the muscle, electrocautery, and reduced muscle tension, and it was our hypothesis that these disturbances caused the arterial anastomoses partially to close down, producing ischaemia in the distal region of the muscle.

To test this idea we used fluorescent microspheres to study the regional blood flow contributed by the two main arterial supplies to the latissimus dorsi muscle in the sheep. We confirmed that both the thoracodorsal artery and the perforating arteries supplied the whole latissimus dorsi muscle, but with oppositely directed gradients. After two weeks of continuous electrical stimulation at 2 Hz, these characteristic gradients were abolished, almost certainly because of increased flow through the anastomotic connections between the two vascular trees [55]. In support of our hypothesis, prestimulation also made the muscle more resistant to surgical disturbance. When untreated muscles were lifted, handled, cooled, and replaced at reduced tension, distal ischaemia was observed, and flow had not recovered significantly five days later. When prestimulated muscles were manipulated in the same way, the reduction in blood flow was smaller, the distal region was no longer selectively affected, and any initial ischaemia was completely reversed by five days [56].

This work suggests that a moderate régime of electrical stimulation, delivered before mobilising the latissimus dorsi muscle, could significantly enhance blood flow to the distal part of the graft from the thoracodorsal artery *via an existing arterial network*. Prestimulation of this kind would also accomplish at least part of the conditioning required for the muscle to perform cardiac levels of work. It would therefore be expected both to improve the viability of the graft and to allow circulatory support to be introduced at an earlier postoperative stage – a great benefit to patients with a limited cardiac reserve.

Improving stimulation protocols for conditioning and activation

The key to cardiac assistance from skeletal muscle is 'conditioning' by electrical stimulation over a period of weeks. This induces the adaptive changes needed if the muscle is to perform cardiac work. Various stimulation patterns have been used for this purpose. In basic scientific studies, continuous stimulation at 10 Hz has been used in rabbits or rats, and a lower frequency, such as 2 Hz, in larger species such as dogs and sheep. The clinical protocol that was introduced with cardiomyoplasty consists of short bursts of stimulation at about 30 Hz, the challenge to the muscle being increased progressively to this level over several weeks. This protocol is far from optimal, for it takes too long and results in the development of slow contractile characteristics, which reduce the power available from the graft and pose problems of synchronisation with the cardiac cycle [38].

We have long argued [17, 39, 45, 46] that it would be far better if conditioning could produce a muscle of the '2A' type, since this would have a highly developed capacity for generating energy via oxidative pathways yet retain fast contractile characteristics. We have shown that such a state can be established, and maintained stably, by conditioning the muscle with a pattern of stimulation that delivers a smaller aggregate amount of impulse activity [18, 28, 53]. Although these muscles appeared to be as fatigue-resistant as muscles that had been completely transformed to the slow oxidative type, they were very much more powerful, the result of both a greater speed of shortening and a higher force-generating capacity, the latter associated with a greater mass of contractile tissue. Clearly a reduction in the total amount of stimulation is highly desirable. How could it be achieved in practice?

One measure would be to replace constant-frequency bursts of impulses, which are conventional but completely unphysiological, with bursts in which the interpulse intervals are varied to produce the greatest force per impulse [22]. Another measure would be to deliver stimulation for only part of the day. For example, assist could be delivered only during specified periods within the 24-hour cycle, or could be restricted to times when a rise in the patient's heart rate signals an increase in demand. Recently this last approach was applied in a clinical situation and it was clearly shown that the contractile speed (and therefore power) of the grafted muscle increased when stimulation was switched from a continuous régime to an intermittent 'on-demand régime' [6].

Another approach to the reduction of total impulse activity is to assist a smaller proportion of cardiac cycles. In fact there are other important reasons for taking this measure, namely the growing evidence that more intensive régimes produce irreversible damage in the graft [19, 31]. This may be related to impaired blood flow in the muscle flap. When a skeletal muscle contracts, the rise in intramuscular pressure may cause its own nutrient blood flow to be arrested or even reversed. Normally forward flow undergoes a compensatory increase during the ensuing relaxation, and mean flow is not affected. If such a muscle is wrapped around the cardiac ventricles and contractions are repeated too frequently, there may not be enough time for the muscle to be reperfused during relaxation. This effect is exacerbated if contraction and relaxation are slowed excessively by over-conditioning. This is an argument in favour of clinical cardiomyoplasty as it was practiced in Russia, where it was normal to use synchronisation ratios between 1:4 and 1:16, apparently to good effect [9]. In a study of the influence of synchronisation ratio in the sheep, Van Doorn and her colleagues found that when the muscle was stimulated on every cardiac cycle there was an increase in thoracodorsal venous lactate concentration and a high incidence of reactive hyperemia; this constitutes clear evidence that a 1:1 régime of stimulation produces partially anaerobic, and therefore unsustainable, working conditions in the muscle [61]. Whether the latissimus dorsi muscle is configured as a cardiomyoplasty wrap or as a skeletal muscle ventricle [62], its long-term viability will be improved if it is not activated more frequently than once in every 4 cardiac cycles. The synchronisation ratio is another variable that could be manipulated according to demand.

Magic bullets?

The loss of mass seen in conventionally conditioned muscles has encouraged some workers to look at pharmacological techniques as an adjunct to stimulation for improving graft function [13, 33]. However, an understanding of the scientific phenomena, resulting in appropriate modifications to the clinical protocol, will often have the desired effect without the additional risks, side-effects, and costs of long-term drug therapy. This is well illustrated by the beneficial effects of reducing the aggregate amount of stimulation delivered to the muscle, as discussed in the preceding section, which produces gains in power and not merely in mass. This said, there may be scope for the temporary use of agents that enhance the viability of the graft by promoting angiogenesis or otherwise preventing ischaemic injury [25, 54].

▪ Conclusion

Harnessing the power of skeletal muscle for cardiac assistance could become a highly effective surgical approach to the treatment of end-stage heart failure. There is no reason why the latissimus dorsi muscle graft should not function permanently in such a role, but much depends on the way in which the muscle is treated before it is mobilised, and on the way it is activated subsequently. It is essential that clinical protocols remain flexible, so that they can accommodate the better understanding of these issues that is beginning to emerge from basic scientific studies.

■ **Acknowledgments.** The author wishes to thank his colleagues in the British Heart Foundation Skeletal Muscle Assist Research Group: Dr. J.C. Jarvis, Mr. E.B.C. Woo, Mr. M. West, Dr. H. Sutherland, Dr. A. Lopez Guajardo, Ms. J. MacDonald, and Mr. J. Blackhurst. The support given to the individuals and the research over the relevant period by The British Heart Foundation, The Beit Memorial Foundation, The G.M. Morrison Trust, and the European Community, is gratefully acknowledged.

■ References

1. Acker MA, Hammond R, Mannion JD, Salmons S, Stephenson LW (1986) An autologous biologic pump motor. J Thorac Cardiovasc Surg 12:733–746
2. Acker MA, Hammond RL, Mannion JD, Salmons S, Stephenson LW (1987) Skeletal muscle as the potential power source for a cardiovascular pump: assessment in vivo. Science 236:324–327
3. Anderson DR, Pochettino A, Hammond RL, Hohenhaus E, Spanta AD, Bridges CR, Jr, Lavine S, Bhan RD, Colson M, Stephenson LW (1991) Autogenously lined skeletal muscle ventricles in circulation. Up to nine months' experience. J Thorac Cardiovasc Surg 101:661–670
4. Anderson WA, Andersen JS, Acker MA, Hammond RL, Chin AJ, Douglas PS, Khalafalla AS, Salmons S, Stephenson LW (1988) Skeletal muscle grafts applied to the heart: a word of caution. Circulation 78 (Suppl III):180–190
5. Capouya ER, Gerber RS, Drinkwater DC, Jr, Pearl JM, Sack JB, Aharon AS, Barthel SW, Kaczer EM, Chang PA, Laks H (1993) Girdling effect of nonstimulated cardiomyoplasty on left ventricular function [see comments]. Ann Thorac Surg 56:867–870
6. Carraro U, Docali G, Barbiero M, Brunazzi C, Gealow K, Casarotto D, Muneretto C (1998) Demand dynamic cardiomyoplasty: improved clinical benefits by non-invasive monitoring of LD flap and long-term tuning of its dynamic contractile characteristics by activity-rest regime. Basic Appl Myol 8:11–15
7. Carroll SM, Carroll CMA, Stremel RW, Heilman SJ, Tobin GR, Barker JH (1997) Vascular delay of the latissimus dorsi muscle: an essential component of cardiomyoplasty. Ann Thorac Surg 63:1034–1040
8. Carroll SM, Heilman SJ, Stremel RW, Tobin GR, Barker JH (1997) Vascular delay improves latissimus dorsi muscle perfusion and muscle function for use in cardiomyoplasty. Plas Reconstr Surg 99:1329–1337
9. Chekanov VS, Krakovsky AA, Bushlenko NS, Riabinina LG, Andreev DB, Shatalov KV, Dubrovsky IA, Pekarsky VV, Akhmedov SD, Trehan N, Shetty K (1994) Cardiomyoplasty. Review of early and late results. Vasc Surg 28:481–488
10. Cheng W, Michele JJ, Spinale FG, Sink JD, Santamore WP (1993) Effects of cardiomyoplasty on biventricular function in canine chronic heart failure. Ann Thorac Surg 55:893–901
11. El Oakley RM, Jarvis JC (1994) Cardiomyoplasty: a critical review of experimental and clinical results. Circulation 90:2085–2090

12. El Oakley RM, Jarvis JC, Barman D, Greenhalgh DL, Currie J, Downham DY, Salmons S, Hooper TL (1995) Factors affecting the integrity of latissimus dorsi muscle grafts: implications for cardiac assistance from skeletal muscle. J Heart Lung Transpl 14:359–365

13. Fritzsche D, Krakor R, Asmussen G, Lange S, Kaufmann A, Zapf P, Melhorn G, Berkei J, Widera R (1994) Effect of an anabolic steroid (Metenolon) on contractile performance of the chronically stimulated latissimus dorsi in sheep. Eur J Cardiothorac Surg 8:214–219

14. Furnary AP, Chachques JC, Moreira LFP, Grunkemeier GL, Swanson JS, Stolf N, Haydar S, Acar C, Starr A, Jatene AD, Carpentier AF (1996) Long-term outcome, survival analysis, and risk stratification of dynamic cardiomyoplasty. J Thorac Cardiovasc Surg 112:1640–1649

15. Grandjean PA, Lori Austin RN, Chan S, Terpestra B, Bourgeois IM (1991) Dynamic cardiomyoplasty: clinical follow-up results. J Cardiac Surg 6:80–88

16. Ianuzzo CD, Ianuzzo SE, Carson N, Feild M, Locke M, Gu J, Anderson WA, Klabunde RE (1996) Cardiomyoplasty: degeneration of the assisting skeletal muscle. J Appl Physiol 80:1205–1213

17. Jarvis JC, Brownson C, Sutherland H, Salmons S (1992) Comparison between the effects of continuous long-term stimulation of rabbit skeletal muscle at 2.5 Hz and 10 Hz. In: Carraro U (ed) Muscle Driven Devices for Cardiac Assistance. Commission of the European Communities, Brussels, pp 29–34

18. Jarvis JC, Sutherland H, Mayne CN, Gilroy SJ, Salmons S (1996) Induction of a fast-oxidative phenotype by chronic muscle stimulation: mechanical and biochemical studies. Am J Physiol 270:C306–312

19. Kalil-Filho R, Bocchi E, Weiss RG, Rosemberg L, Bacal F, Moreira LFP, Stolf NAG, Magalhães AAC, Belotti G, Jatene A, Pileggi F (1994) Magnetic resonance imaging evaluation of chronic changes in latissimus dorsi cardiomyoplasty. Circulation 90:II 102–II 106

20. Kantrowitz A, McKinnon W (1959) The experimental use of the diaphragm as an auxiliary myocardium. Surgical Forum 9:266–268

21. Kass DA, Baughman KL, Pak PH, Cho PW, Levin HR, Gardner TJ, Halperin HR, Tsitlik JE, Acker MA (1995) Reverse remodeling from cardiomyoplasty in human heart failure. External constraint versus active assist. Circulation 91:2314–2318

22. Kwende MMN, Jarvis JC, Salmons S (1995) The input-output relationships of skeletal muscle. Proc Roy Soc Lond Ser B 261:193–201

23. Le Tissier P, Stoye JP, Takeuchi Y, Patience C, Weiss RA (1997) Two sets of human-tropic pig retrovirus. Nature 389:681–682

24. Lucas CMHB, van der Veen FH, Cheriex EC, Lorusso R, Havenith M, Penn OCKM, Wellens HJJ (1993) Long-term follow-up (12 to 35 weeks) after dynamic cardiomyoplasty. J Amer Coll Cardiol 22:758–767

25. Mannion JD, Blood V, Bailey W, Bauer TL, Magno MG, DiMeo F, Epple A, Spinale FG (1996) The effect of basic fibroblast growth factor on the blood flow and morphologic features of a latissimus dorsi cardiomyoplasty. J Thorac Cardiovasc Surg 111:19–28

26. Mannion JD, Hammond RL, Stephenson LW (1986) Canine latissimus dorsi hydraulic pouches: potential for left ventricular assistance. J Thorac Cardiovasc Surg 91:534–544

27. Mannion JD, Velchik M, Hammond R, Alavi A, Mackler T, Duckett S, Staum M, Hurwitz S, Brown W, Stephenson LW (1989) Effects of collateral blood vessel ligation and electrical conditioning on blood flow in dog latissimus dorsi muscle. J Surg Res 47:332–340

28. Mayne CN, Sutherland H, Jarvis JC, Gilroy SJ, Craven AJ, Salmons S (1996) Induction of a fast-oxidative phenotype by chronic muscle stimulation: histochemical and metabolic studies. Am J Physiol 270:C313–320

29. McCarthy PM (1996) Ventricular remodelling: hype or hope? Nature Medicine 2:859–860

30. Moreira LFP, Bocchi EA, Stolf NAG, Bellotti G, Jatene AD (1996) Dynamic cardiomyoplasty in the treatment of dilated cardiomyopathy – current results and perspectives. J Cardiac Surg 11:207–216

31. Moreira LFP, Bocchi EA, Stolf NAG, Pileggi F, Jatene AD (1993) Current expectations in dynamic cardiomyoplasty. Ann Thorac Surg 55:299–303

32. Oh JH, Badhwar V, Chiu RC-J (1996) Mechanisms of dynamic cardiomyoplasty – current concepts. J Cardiac Surg 11:194–199

33. Petrou M, Wynne D, Boheler K, Yacoub M (1995) Clenbuterol induces hypertrophy of the latissimus dorsi muscle and heart in the rat with molecular and phenotypic changes. Circulation 92:II483–II489

34. Pochettino A, Anderson DR, Hammond RL, Salmons S, Stephenson LW (1991) Skeletal muscle ventricles. Sem Thorac Cardiovasc Surg 3:154–159

35. Radermecker MA, Triffaux M, Fissette J, Limet R (1992) Anatomical rationale for use of the latissimus dorsi flap during the cardiomyoplasty operation. Surg Radiol Anat 14:5–10

36. Salmons PH, Salmons S (1992) Psychological costs of high-tech heart surgery (guest editorial). Br J Hosp Med 48:707–709

37. Salmons S (1975) On the feasibility of using diaphragm muscle as a myocardial substitute. Med Biol Eng 13:608–609

38. Salmons S (1992) Optimizing the benefits of cardiomyoplasty. Br J Hosp Med 49:137

39. Salmons S (1994) Exercise, stimulation and type transformation of skeletal muscle. Int J Sports Med 15:136–141

40. Salmons S (1997) Damage in functional grafts of skeletal muscle. In: Muscle Damage. Salmons S (ed) Oxford University Press, Oxford, pp 215–233

41. Salmons S, Henriksson J (1981) The adaptive response of skeletal muscle to increased use. Muscle Nerve 4:94–105

42. Salmons S, Jarvis JC (1990) Cardiomyoplasty: the basic issues. Cardiac Chronicle 4:1–7

43. Salmons S, Jarvis JC (1991) Cardiomyoplasty: a look at the fundamentals. In: Carpentier A, Chachques JC, Grandjean PA (eds) Cardiomyoplasty. Futura Publishing Company, Inc., Mount Kisco, NY, pp 3–17

44. Salmons S, Jarvis JC (1992) Cardiac assistance from skeletal muscle: a critical appraisal of the various approaches. Br Heart J 68:333–338

45. Salmons S, Jarvis JC (1993) Measuring, estimating and preserving skeletal muscle power for cardiac assistance. In: Proceedings of the 4th Vienna International Workshop on Functional Electrostimulation: Basics, Technology, Clinical Application. Vienna, ISBN 3-900928-02-9, pp 26–29

46. Salmons S, Jarvis JC (1995) Educating skeletal muscle to do cardiac work. In: Lewis T, Graham TR, Frazier OH, Hill JD, Pennington DG, Salmons S (eds) Mechanical Circulatory Support. Edward Arnold, London, pp 259–266

47. Salmons S, Sréter FA (1976) Significance of impulse activity in the transformation of skeletal muscle type. Nature 263:30–34

48. Salmons S, Tang ATM, Jarvis JC, Degens H, Hastings M, Hooper TL (1998) Morphological and functional evidence, and clinical importance, of vascular anastomoses in the latissimus dorsi muscle of the sheep. J Anat 193:93–104

49. Shortland A, Black RA, Jarvis JC, Salmons S (1996) Factors influencing vortex development in a model of a skeletal muscle ventricle. Artif Org 20:1026–1033

50. Shortland AP, Black RA, Jarvis JC, Henry FS, Iudicello F, Collins MW, Salmons S (1996) Formation and travel of vortices in model ventricles: application to the design of skeletal muscle ventricles. J Biomech 29:503–511

51. Shortland AP, Black RA, Jarvis JC, Salmons S (1996) A novel video technique for visualizing flow structures in cardiovascular models. J Biomech 29:239–244

52. Shortland AP, Iudicello F, Black RA, Jarvis JC, Henry FS, Collins MW, Salmons S (1997) Physical and numerical simulation of blood flow within a skeletal muscle ventricle. In: Carpentier AF, Chachques JC, Grandjean PA (eds) Cardiac Bioassist. Futura Publishing Co. Inc., Armonk, New York, pp 567–573

53. Sutherland H, Jarvis JC, Kwende MMN, Gilroy SJ, Salmons S (1998) The dose-related response of rabbit fast muscle to long-term low-frequency stimulation. Muscle Nerve 21:1632–1646

54. Tang ATM, Geraghty P, Dascombe MJ, Jarvis JC, Salmons S, Hooper TL (1998) Nitroglycerine reduces neutrophil activation and acute damage in latissimus dorsi muscle grafts. Ann Thorac Surg 66:2015–2021

55. Tang ATM, Jarvis JC, Hooper TL, Salmons S (1998) Observation and basis of improved blood flow to the distal latissimus dorsi muscle: a case for electrical stimulation prior to grafting. Cardiovasc Res 40:131–137

56. Tang ATM, Jarvis JC, Hooper TL, Salmons S (1999) Cardiomyoplasty: the benefits of electrical prestimulation of the latissimus dorsi muscle in situ. Ann Thorac Surg 68:46–51

57. Tang G, Hooper T (1997) Dynamic cardiomyoplasty. Br J Hosp Med 57:329–332

58. Thomas GA, Baciewicz FA, Jr, Hammond RL, Greer KA, Lu H, Bastion S, Jindal P, Stephenson LW (1998) Power output of pericardium-lined skeletal muscle ventricles, left ventricular apex to aorta configuration: up to eight months in circulation. J Thorac Cardiovasc Surg 116:1029–1042

59. Thomas GA, Isoda S, Hammond RL, Lu HP, Nakajima H, Nakajima HO, Greer K, Gilroy SJ, Salmons S, Stephenson LW (1996) Pericardium-lined skeletal muscle ventricles: up to two years' in-circulation experience. Ann Thorac Surg 62:1698–1706

60. Trainini JC (1999) Dynamic cardiomyoplasty and aortomyoplasty: the Buenos Aires experience. Basic Appl Myol 8:413–418

61. van Doorn CAM, Bhabra MS, Hopkinson DN, Barman D, Cranley JJ, Hooper TL (1996) Latissimus dorsi muscle blood flow during synchronized contraction – implications for cardiomyoplasty. Ann Thorac Surg 61:603–609

62. van Doorn CAM, Degens H, Bhabra MS, Till CBW, Shaw TE, Jarvis JC, Salmons S, Hooper TL (1997) Intramural blood flow of skeletal muscle ventricles functioning as aortic counterpulsators. Ann Thorac Surg 64:86–93

Author's address:

Professor Stanley Salmons
Department of Human Anatomy and Cell Biology
New Medical School, Ashton Street
University of Liverpool
Liverpool L69 3GE, U.K.
E-mail: s.salmons@liverpool.ac.uk

CHAPTER **5** **Cardiomyoplasty in chronic heart failure: the Paris Experience**

J. C. CHACHQUES and A. CARPENTIER

■ Introduction

Congestive cardiac failure is caused by a decrease in myocardial contractility due to mechanical overload or by an initial defect in the myocardial fiber. The alteration in diastolic function is inextricably linked with the pathophysiology of cardiac insufficiency. Despite a widely varying and diverse etiology of congestive cardiac failure, the pathophysiology is to a great extent constant. The predominant factor is the alteration of myocardial contractility. This contractility defect causes an elevation of the ventricular wall tension resulting in a progressive decline in the contractile state of the myocardial fibers [18, 19].

The aim of cardiomyoplasty (CMP) is to restore or enhance the myocardial contractility using the patient's latissimus dorsi muscle (LDM) which is wrapped around the ventricles and electrostimulated in synchrony with the contractions of the heart. This technique has been used world-wide in clinical medicine on more than 1500 patients of which 112 were treated at Broussais Hospital [2, 3, 8, 9].

The biological support of this operation consists of chronic muscle electrostimulation which induces a physiological adaptation of skeletal muscle to cardiac work ("myocardization of the LDM"). The metabolism of the rapid glycolytic fatigue-sensitive muscle fibers (type II) are transformed into slow oxidative fatigue-resistant muscle fibers (type I) [1, 6].

The electronic stimulation materials consist of an implantable Cardio-Myostimulator, muscle stimulation electrodes, and systole detection electrodes which allow the synchronization of muscle contractions to the heart beat. In order to imitate the duration of a systolic contraction, the skeletal muscle should be electrostimulated using train impulses with a duration close to the ventricular ejection time span.

■ Indications

CMP is recommended to patients suffering from severe chronic cardiac deficiency. The ischemic myocardial deficiency (patients presenting successive infarctions or one largely extended) as well as dilated cardiomyopa-

Table 1. Criteria for cardiomyoplasty patient selection

Indications
- ▓ Indiopathic dilated or ischemic cardiomyopathies
- ▓ Severe heart failure (but not yet end-stage, i.e., patient has some cardiac reserve: radioisotopic LV ejection fraction > 15%; peak VO$_2$ > 10 ml/kg/min)
- ▓ Intact left latissimus dorsi muscle with preserved force
- ▓ Adult (fully grown)

Contraindications
- ▓ Severe mitral valve regurgitation
- ▓ Preoperative dependence on intravenous inotropes of intra-aortic balloon counterpulsation
- ▓ Primary hypertrophic or restrictive cardiomyopathy
- ▓ Cardiac cachexia

thies (generally of unknown origin) are considered to be indications for CMP. Hypertrophic or obstructive cardiomyopathies, however, are excluding factors for CMP (Table 1).

The time to perform a CMP can be concluded from the postoperative results. The hemodynamic advantage of the CMP is only achieved after a delay of several weeks corresponding to the adaptation period of the LDM to its new cardiac assistance function. Therefore, the residual myocardial function has to be taken into account in patient selection.

▓ Surgical technique

An oblique incision is made in the postero-lateral region of the thorax in order to dissect the left LDM (Fig. 1). Its vascular-nervous pedicule, originating from the axillary region, is carefully preserved. After implantation of two stimulation electrodes (Fig. 2), a window is created in the thoracic wall by partial resection of the second rib. The LDM is then transferred through the window to the inside of the thorax [7].

The patient is placed in the decubitus dorsal position. Extracorporeal circulation is technically not necessary during this type of surgery. A medial sternotomy allows one to open the pericardium and expose the heart. The LDM is fixed around the ventricles. The two most frequent intraoperative complications during the heart wrapping are malignant ventricular arrhythmias and hemodynamic deterioration resulting from manipulation of the dilated heart. To avoid these complications, the LDM is passed posteriorly around the ventricles without lifting the heart. This maneuver is performed using two long curved hemostatic clamps, afterwards the LDM is fixed with interrupted sutures to the pericardium. The wrapping is completed by fixing the anterior part of the LDM to itself (in a pocket fashion) and to a pericardial flap, tailored from the right edge of the pericardiotomy. Care is taken to ensure that the heart is not subjected to excess tension or compression from the LDM wrapping (Fig. 3).

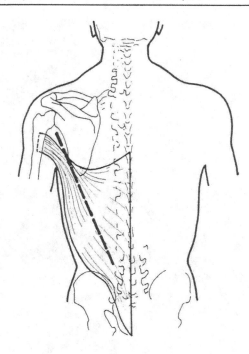

Fig. 1. Skin incision for LDM dissection and transposition into the chest

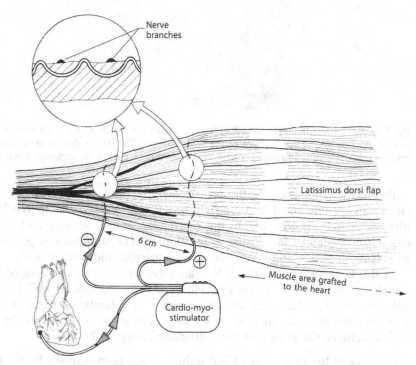

Fig. 2. Two intramuscular pacing electrodes are implanted into the proximal part of the LDM

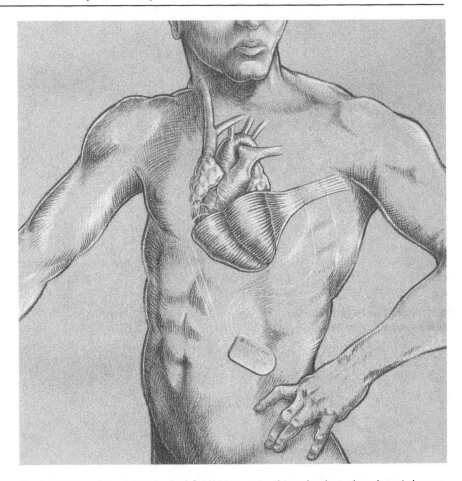

Fig. 3. Cardiomyoplasty technique: the left LDM is transposed into the chest through a window created by resecting the anterior segment of the 2nd rib (5 cm). The LDM is then wrapped arround both ventricles. Sensing and pacing electrodes are connected to an implantable cardiomyostimulator

Before the completion of the ventricular wrapping, one or two sensing electrodes are implanted into the right or left ventricular walls, to synchronize the muscle contractions to the ventricular systole. Sensing and impedance are verified to assure proper positioning. The stimulator is placed in an epigastric pocket and connected to the muscular and cardiac leads.

In the CMP technique, the LDM can serve as an enhancement of the ventricular systole in ischemic or dilated cardiomyopathies, as well as partial myocardial replacement after resection of a voluminous aneurysm or an extensive tumor. In the latter cases a pericardial patch is used as the interface between the LDM and the ventricular cavity [4, 7].

The choice of the LDM in the CMP technique has been justified by the following anatomical and physiological conditions:

■ its proximity to the heart,
■ the extent of muscular mass with the possibility of intrathoracic transposition while keeping the vascular-nervous pedicule intact,
■ absence of important functional sequelae at the level of the superior
  limbs after removal of the LDM.

The third condition has also been observed by plastic surgeons who frequently use the LDM to reconstruct the thoracic wall, the cervical region
or the upper limb.

■ Electrostimulation of the heart and skeletal muscles

Cardiac and skeletal muscles differ in their structure and their response to
electrostimulation. The depolarization of a single cell of the myocardium
induces an action potential that travels through the whole cardiac muscle
which, in turn, leads to an instantaneous contraction of atria and ventricles. Only one single impulse above a given threshold is needed to start
this process.

Skeletal muscle also shows electrophysiological differences. The amplitude and duration of the contractions can be influenced by stimulation
parameters. The modulation of the amplitude and/or of the impulse size
modifies the number of motor units activated (spatial recruitment)
whereas the number of impulses and the duration between each impulse
modifies the excitation frequency of motor units (temporal recruitment). A
series of impulse produces, therefore, a contraction, variable in force,
which is supported in time by an additional effect [1, 3] (Fig. 4).

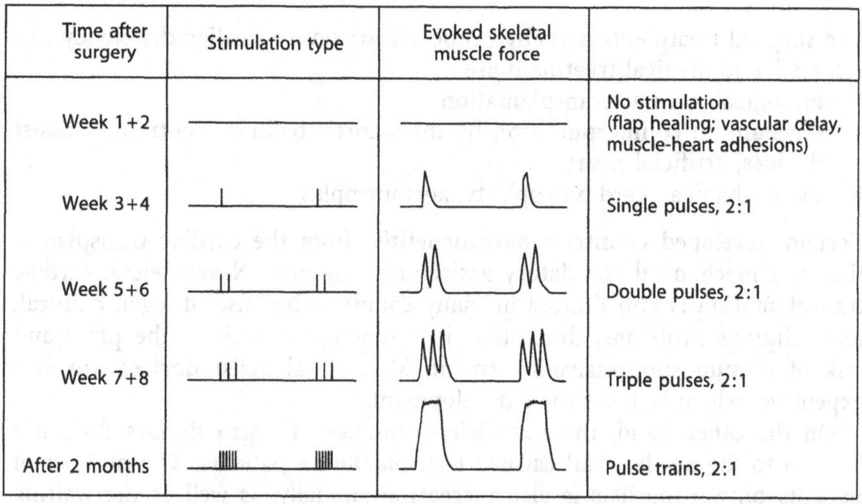

Time after surgery	Stimulation type	Evoked skeletal muscle force	
Week 1+2			No stimulation (flap healing; vascular delay, muscle-heart adhesions)
Week 3+4			Single pulses, 2:1
Week 5+6			Double pulses, 2:1
Week 7+8			Triple pulses, 2:1
After 2 months			Pulse trains, 2:1

Fig. 4. Post-operative stimulation protocol. The LDM is progressively electrostimulated after the 2nd
postoperative week. The final heart to muscle ratio is 2:1. (From [6])

The electrical activation of skeletal muscles is known in other clinical applications: in the treatment of respiratory paralysis (stimulation of the diaphragm or more precisely the phrenic nerve); in colorectal surgery (surgical creation of a neosphincter using the gracilis muscle, electrostimulation of this muscle allows an efficient continence); in urology (vesicomyoplasty and neosphincter); in the correction of scoliosis (stimulation of the paravertebrae muscles); in the treatment of paraplegia (stimulation of inferior limb muscles); and in orthopedia (rehabilitation of the musculature after prolonged inactivation).

■ Action mechanisms

CMP improves cardiac performance by several mechanisms:
■ Enhancement of the ventricular systolic ejection (an effect comparable to a heart massage)
■ Limiting cardiac dilatation
■ Ventricular wall stress reduction
■ Ventricular cavity remodeling

CMP leads to an increase in ventricular mass by adding a new contractile muscular wall which allows, in turn, the reestablishments of the ratio between the mass and the ventricular diameter in dilated cardiomyopathies [11, 15, 17].

■ Place of cardiomyoplasty

The surgical treatments actually proposed for severe cardiac deficiency unresponsive to medical treatment are
■ biological: cardiac transplantation
■ mechanical: counterpulsation by intra-aortic balloon, ventricular assist devices, artificial heart
■ biomechanical: cardiomyoplasty, aortomyoplasty

Certain developed countries have benefited from the cardiac transplantation and mechanical circulatory assistance programs. Nevertheless, cardiac transplantation is still limited in many countries because of legal, cultural, and religious problems, difficulties in follow-up, as well as the price and risk of immunosuppressive treatment. Mechanical assist devices are also expensive, which reduces their development.

On the other hand, the insufficient number of organ donors does not face up to the needs of all cardiac transplantation patients. The number of patients on waiting lists is also increasing annually, as well as the waiting period. Therefore, it is logical to propose to these patients, with a high risk of mortality, other therapeutic possibilities [18, 19].

CMP has the advantage of constituting a complete implantable cardiac assistance system which is entirely biocompatible. Recent progress in biology and skeletal muscle electrostimulation has demonstrated that the latter could transform the muscle to be resistant to fatigue and, hence, become an important source of circulatory assistance.

The biomechanical system is a combination of cardiac and plastic surgery with biomedical engineering. Its aim is to prolong and improve the quality of life of patients who suffer from severe chronic cardiac deficiency and who are unresponsive to medical treatment. In CMP, the musculature of the same subject is used which excludes the risk of rejection and, therefore, eliminates immunosuppressive treatment. The clinical follow-up is simple since the function of the cardiomyostimulator is essentially checked. Long-term results are encouraging, particularly since the indications are more precisely identified [4, 9, 12–14].

■ Cardiomyoplasty: clinical experience

The management of patients with end stage heart failure is a daily challenge in cardiac surgery. Cardiac transplantation and mechanical assist devices do not cover all the needs.

■ **Patient population:** Between 1985 and 1999, 112 patients aged 15 to 72 years (mean 51 years) were operated in our institution. All patients presented a severe cardiac deficiency refractory to maximal pharmacological therapy; 86 were in NYHA class III and 26 in class IV. Ejection fraction averaged 17%, EDLV volume 178 ± 31 ml/m^2. The cause of heart failure was ischemia in 59 patients, dilated cardiomyopathy in 46 patients, and ventricular tumors in 7 patients. Associated pathology (pulmonary hypertension, diabetes, etc.) was present in 60%. The technique has evolved from "open fixation" (58 patients), to "non-suture wrapping" (41 patients), to "mini-invasive technique" (13 patients). Two-stage operations in high risk patients with mitral valve insufficiency or severe arrhythmia were performed in 6 patients. Associated procedures were necessary in 24 patients (CABG = 14, valve = 10).

■ **Results:** Hospital mortality was 53% between 1985–1987, 13% between 1988–1997, and 8% since the introduction of mini-invasive techniques. Actuarial survival at 10 years was 70% for preop class III patients and 28% for class IV patients. Average NYHA class was 3.3 preop and 1.4 postop. Nine patients required transplantation. Hemodynamic investigations in the survivors showed significant improvement in ejection fraction (21% to 31%) and cardiac index (1.9 to 2.8 L/mn/m^2).

The clinical evaluation and the postoperative studies show that CMP is an efficient technique to assist chronic patients who suffer from severe cardiac deficiency. The technique allows a functional improvement of the patient's capacity during exercise, as well as a decrease in medication. In operated patients a decrease was noted in deterioration of their state which would have required hospitalization.

The quality of life of the patients, evaluated every six months postoperatively by questionnaire, significantly improved since most patients had increased their daily and social activities and 62% had started working again. The CMP results improved through experience, through rigorous patient selection, through progress in the operation technique, and through improved postoperative care. The postoperative course was often critical (30% low cardiac output syndrome), particularly in ischemic etiology.

▪ **Conclusion:** Cardiomyoplasty has been associated with better results due to technical improvements, the most significant being mini-invasive techniques, the latest, the use of growth factors to enhance muscle vascularization. Cardiac transplantation is technically feasible after a CMP. Risk factors have been identified resulting in more precise indications, a lower hospital mortality, and a wider use of this operation.

▪ Perspectives

Electrophysiological treatments associated with CMP

The patients who have been subjected to a CMP, suffering from ischemic or severe idiopathic cardiomyopathy, present a great risk for ventricular arrhythmias which is potentially responsible for the occurrence of sudden death. At the same time, electrical and mechanical asynchronisms between the ventricles are frequently observed in these patients. In recent clinical cases, CMP has been associated with an implantable defibrillator or biventricular stimulation (multisite pacing). The very positive results obtained foresee an important expansion of these associated techniques.

Video-assisted mini-invasive techniques

In cardiovascular surgery, recent clinical experiences (in the case of coronary and valve surgery) have demonstrated the interest of using mini-invasive techniques. Fundamentally, the advantage for the patient is aesthetic, however, rehabilitation is much quicker, and it avoids the risk of complications from a sternotomy. Since October 1997, thirteen CMPs have been carried out in our department using reduced access routes with very encouraging results [10].

Growth factors and cardiomyoplasty

The LDM which is fixed around the heart can cause cellular alterations due to the dissection, intrathoracic transposition, and electrostimulation.

Growth factors (agents which increase cell proliferation and induce cell migration) could have a beneficial effect on muscle fibers. In our department, we have started a research study to evaluate the action of growth factors on a CMP model: basic fibroblast growth factor (bFGF), vascular endothelial growth factor (VEGF), as well as heparin sulphate (RGTA). The use of these factors improve the development of the collateral circulation between the heart, the LDM, and the mediastin structures by stimulation of angiogenesis.

Cellular cardiomyoplasty

Cellular cardiomyoplasty is an approach to implant cells and grow new muscle fibers in the damaged myocardium that may potentially contribute to the contractile performance of the heart.

Since cardiomyocytes cannot regenerate after ischemia, the injury is irreversible. Therefore, the aim of cellular cardiomyoplasty is the repair of injured myocardium by cell transplantation, either in ischemic or idiopathic cardiomyopathies. Two types of cells have mainly been used for this purpose:

■ fetal cardiomyocytes, an approach which presents two major disadvantages:
  - the availability of embryonic (or fetal) tissue is limited.
  - an immunosuppressive treatment is required after implantation of cardiomyocytes.
■ autologous myoblasts obtained from skeletal muscles of the same individual. The satellite cells or myoblasts can be obtained in large quantities, furthermore the autologous implantation does not cause any immunological rejection problems. Cellular cardiomyoplasty research is at a developing stage in our department. The main questions are how satellite cells integrate into myocardiac tissue and whether the cells can provide an improvement in contractile force [16].

■ References

1. Arpesella G, Carraro U, Mikus PM, Dozza F, Lombardi P, Marinelli G, Zampieri S, El Messlemani AH, Rossini K, Pierangeli A (1998) Activity-rest stimulation of latissimus dorsi for cardiomyoplasty. Ann Thorac Surg 66:1983–1990
2. Carpentier A, Chachques JC (1985) Myocardial substitution with a stimulated skeletal muscle: first successful clinical case. Lancet 8440:1267
3. Carpentier A, Chachques JC, Grandjean P (eds) (1991) Cardiomyoplasty. Futura Publishing, New York, pp 1–280
4. Carpentier A, Chachques JC, Acar C, Relland J, Mihaileanu S, Bensasson D, Kieffer JP, Guibourt P, Tournay D, Roussin I, Grandjean PA (1993) Dynamic cardiomyoplasty at seven years. J Thorac Cardiovasc Surg 106:42–54
5. Carpentier A, Chachques JC, Grandjean P (eds) (1997) Cardiac Bioassist. Futura Publishing, New York, pp 1–632

6. Chachques JC, Grandjean PA, Schwartz K, Mihaileanu S, Fardeau M, Swynghedauw B, Fontaliran F, Romero N, Wisnewsky C, Perier P, Chauvaud S, Bourgeois I, Carpentier A (1988) Effect of latissimus dorsi dynamic cardiomyoplasty on ventricular function. Circulation 78 (Suppl 3):203–216
7. Chachques JC, Grandjean PA, Carpentier A (1989) Latissimus dorsi dynamic cardiomyoplasty. Ann Thorac Surg 47:600–604
8. Chachques JC, Berrebi A, Hernigou A, Cohen-Solal A, Lavergne T, Marino JP, D'Attellis N, Bensasson D, Carpentier A (1997) Study of muscular and ventricular function in dynamic cardiomyoplasty: a ten year follow up. J Heart Lung Transplant 16:854–868
9. Chachques JC, Marino JP, Lajos P, Zegdi R, D'Attellis N, Fornes P, Fabiani JN, Carpentier A (1997) Dynamic cardiomyoplasty: clinical follow-up at twelve years. Eur J Cardio-Thorac Surg 12:560–568
10. Chachques JC, Zakine G, D'Attellis N, Carpentier A (1998) Minimally invasive video-assisted cardiomyoplasty. Basic Appl Myol 8:77
11. Chen FY, deGuzman BJ, Aklog L, Lautz DB, Ahmad RM, Laurence RG, Couper GS, Cohn LH, McMahon TA (1996) Decreased myocardial oxygen consumption indices in dynamic cardiomyoplasty. Circulation 94; (Suppl II):239–244
12. Furnary AP, Chachques JC, Moreira LFP, Grunkemeier GL, Swanson JS, Stolf N, Haydar S, Acar C, Starr A, Jatene AD, Carpentier AF (1996) Long term outcome, survival analysis and risk stratification of dynamic cardiomyoplasty. J Thorac Cardiovasc Surg 112:1640–1650
13. Furnary AP, Jessup M, Moreira LFP, for the American Cardiomyoplasty Group (1996) Multicenter trial of dynamic cardiomyoplasty for chronic heart failure. J Am Coll Cardiol 28:1175–1180
14. Lorusso R, Milan E, Volterrani M, Giubbini R, Van der Veen FH, Schreuder JJ, Picchioni A, Alfieri O (1997) Cardiomyoplasty as an isolated procedure to treat refractory heart failure. Eur J Cardio-Thoracic Surg 11:363–372
15. Patel HJ, Lankford EB, Polidori DJ, Pilla JJ, Plappert T, Sutton MSJ, Acker MA (1997) Dynamic cardiomyoplasty: its chronic and acute effects on the failing heart. J Thorac Cardiovasc Surg 114:169–178
16. Rajnoch C, Chachques JC, Lajos P, Fornes P, Mirochnik N, Fabiani JN, Carpentier A (1998) Cell therapy for heart failure. Cardiovasc Surg 6 (Suppl 1):3
17. Schreuder JJ, Van der Veen FH, Ven der Velde ET, Delahaye F, Alfieri O, Jegaden O, Lorusso R, Jansen JR, Hoeksel SA, Finet G, Volterrani M, Kaulbach HG, Baan J, Wellens HJJ (1997) Left ventricular pressure-volume relationships before and after cardiomyoplasty in patients with heart failure. Circulation 96:2978–2986
18. Yamaguchi A, Ino T, Adachi H, Murata S, Kamio H, Okada M, Tsuboi J (1998) Left ventricular volume predicts postoperative course in patients with ischemic cardiomyopathy. Ann Thorac Surg 65:434–8
19. Zannad F, Briancon S, Juilliere Y, Mertes PM, Villemot JP, Alla F, Virion JM, and the EPICAL Investigators (1999) Incidence, clinical and etiologic features, and outcomes of advanced chronic heart failure: the EPICAL study. J Am Coll Cardiol 33:734–742

Author's address:

Juan C. Chachques, MD, PhD
Department of Cardiovascular Surgery
Broussais Hospital
96, rue Didot
75014 Paris, France
E-mail: j.chachques@brs.ap-hop-paris.fr

CHAPTER **6** **Biomechanical hearts
in aorta-descendens position –
operative procedure and volumetry
in adult goats***

N. W. Guldner, P. Klapproth, M. Grossherr,
and H. H. Sievers

Background

Desirable properties of skeletal muscle for cardiac assistance include fatique resistance and powerful mechanical performance. Current clinical application of nonfatigable muscle was limited due to the profound power loss after electrical conditioning. In long-term investigations, skeletal muscle ventricles (SMVs) were performed around an elastic intrathoracic elastic training device. SMVs were treated over several months by a threefold approach in order to achieve nonfatigable and powerful skeletal muscle ventricles (SMVs) by a combination of electrical conditioning, dynamic training against systemic load, and pharmacological support with clenbuterol. SMVs treated in that way became powerful, as demonstrated elsewhere. They were expected to become effective as muscular blood pumps performed in a one-step operation and trained within circulation. This autologous muscular blood pump with a stabilizing inlay, performed in a one-step operation and trained within the circulation, is defined as a biomechanical heart (BMH). Methods for an operative procedure and stroke volume determination are described below.

Methods

The operative procedure is performed in adult Boer goats under general anesthesia. Dissection of the latissimus dorsi muscle is shown in Fig. 1. Myoelectrodes are placed wavelike around the branches of the nervus thoracodorsalis. The threshold of the muscle is determined by electrical stimulation. From a double layered muscular tube of latissimus dorsi muscle, a skeletal muscle ventricle is placed around a silicone-polyurethan inlay and inserted into the thorax after partial resection of the 3rd and 4th rib. Through an inferior thoracotomy, the vascular prostheses from the ventricular inlay of the BMH are anastomosed with the descending aorta end-to-side (Fig. 2). The aorta is ligated totally between the two anastomo-

---

* Presented at the conference as a video.

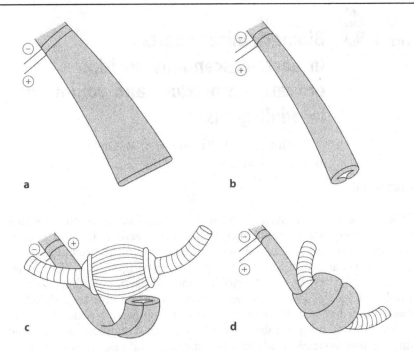

Fig. 1. Operative procedure constructing a BMH with the latissimus dorsi muscle

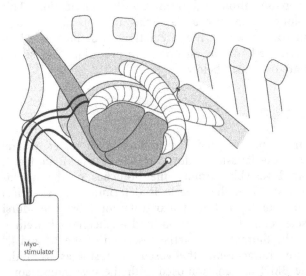

Fig. 2. Topography of a biomechanical heart in the aorta-descendens position in a goat

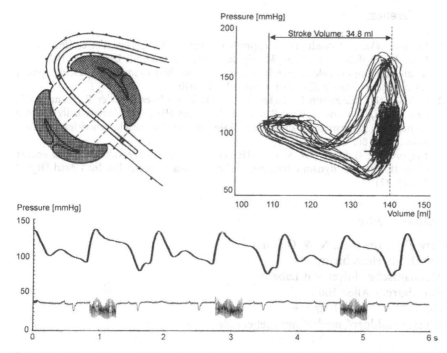

Fig. 3. Volumetry within a BMH by the conductance-catheter-method (*top*). ECG with stimulation bursts and pressure trace from a peripheral artery with BMH contractions in 1:2 mode (*bottom*)

ses. A myocardial sensing electrode is placed and connected with a myostimulator to trigger muscle contractions in the sense of counterpulsation. Pump function of the BMH after several weeks of a dynamic training is demonstrated by arterial blood pressure, ventriculography, and by means of a conductance catheter resulting in pressure-volume loops (Fig. 3).

▪ Results

A BMH was constructed by a latissimus dorsi muscle of 330 g and trained with clenbuterol support within the circulation in an adults male Boere. Evaluated by the conductance catheter method, this BMH with a beat frequency of 40 per minute and a stroke volume of 35 ml pumped 1.4 liter blood per minute continuously after 132 days of training.

▪ Conclusion

A biomechanical heart is performed in a one-step procedure and trained within the circulation. It showed to be hemodynamically relevant and is expected to become clinic practicable for the treatment of end-stage heart failure.

■ References

1. Guldner NW, Eichstaedt HC, Klapproth P, Tilmans MHJ, Thuaudet S, Umbrain V, Ruck K, Wyffels E, Bruyland M, Sigmund M, Messmer BJ, Bardos P (1994) Dynamic training of skeletal muscle ventricles. A method to increase muscular power for cardiac assistance. Circulation 89(3):1032–1040
2. Guldner NW, Klapproth P, Fischer T, Rumpel E, Büchner I, Keller R, Klempien R, Krischer H, Thuaudet S, Noel R, Kuppe H, Sievers HH (1997) Functionally adapted stimulation patterns for a dynamic training of skelatal muscle ventricles in adults goats. BAM 8(1):67–72
3. Klapproth P, Guldner NW, Sievers HH (1997) Stroke volume validation and energy evaluation for the dynamic training of skeletal muscle ventricles. Int J Artif Organs 20:313–321

Author's address:

Priv. Doz. Dr. med. N. W. Guldner
Klinik für Herzchirurgie
Medizinische Universität Lübeck
Ratzeburger Allee 160
D-23538 Lübeck, Germany
E-mail: Guldner@medinf.mu-luebeck.de

CHAPTER **7** **Geometrical considerations in (reverse) remodeling**

CH. J. F. HOLUBARSCH

▪ Introduction

Chronic heart failure results from a number of different diseases. Myocardial infraction, myocarditis, dilative cardiomyopathy, pressure- and/or volume-overload may lead – sooner or later – to left ventricular dilation. This change in left ventricular dimensions is associated with an increase in left ventricular (LV) muscle mass and subtle molecular alterations which per se may contribute to decreased myocardial performance. The sum of these macroscopic, cellular, and subcellular alterations is called LV remodeling.

Due to application of modern medical therapy for chronic heart failure, especially angiotensin-converting enzyme (ACE) inhibitors and beta-adrenoceptor blockers (β-blockers), it became evident that improvement of *both* symptoms *and* survival is accompanied by a reversal remodeling, i. e., a decrease in end-diastolic volume and an increase in ejection fraction [10, 21, 22, 28].

In the last decade, new surgical techniques have been developed for dilated ventricles and heart failure with the goal of decreasing left ventricular size and unloading left ventricular myocardium [2, 9, 18, 30]. As a result, the working conditions for the myocardium are chronically changed, which may also have energetic consequences. In this contribution, left ventricular geometrical parameters are analyzed in 19 subjects with normal LV geometry and function as well as in 37 patients with dilated cardiomyopathy NYHA class II–III with enlarged ventricles and moderately to severely reduced left ventricular function. In addition, myocardial oxygen consumption was measured invasively so that myocardial efficiency could be analyzed. The following results were obtained:

- ▪ The mechanical parameter which correlated best with myocardial oxygen consumption was the systolic stress-time integral.
- ▪ The stress-time integral was 42% greater in dilated cardiomyopathy as compared to the controls.
- ▪ Myocardial efficiency correlated inversely and significantly to end-diastolic LV volume.
- ▪ The decrease in efficiency can be explained on the basis of human cardiac muscle experiments in which isotonic shortening contractions were allowed so that myocardial work could be analyzed as a function of afterload.

▦ Methods

Patients

Fifty-six patients were enrolled in the study. All patients were in sinus rhythm. Nineteen patients had normal left ventricles and normal coronary arteries. These patients underwent heart catheterization and coronary angiography because of a history of atypical chest pain in order to exclude heart disease with certainty. The mean age was 50.4 ± 9.7 years. Thirteen were male; six were female. Thirty-seven patients suffered from idiopathic dilated cardiomyopathy. Patients with mitral valve regurgitation exceeding angiographic degree 1+ [11] were excluded from the study. Thirty were male, seven were female. The mean age was 49.4 ± 9.8 years. Seventeen patients were in NYHA class III; 20 patients were in class II. The diagnosis of dilated cardiomyopathy was defined by increased left ventricular end-diastolic volume (>220 ml) and reduced left ventricular ejection fraction ($<55\%$) in the absence of coronary or valvular heart disease or a history of arterial hypertension.

Study protocol

All patients had given written, informed consent prior to cardiac catheterization. The study protocol was reviewed and approved by the Ethical Committee of the University Clinics of Freiburg.

Cardiac catheterization was performed in the morning after fasting for more than 14 hours. All medications including digitoxin, nitrates, calcium channel blockers, antiarrhythmogenic drugs (propafenone and flecainide) were withdrawn at least 48 hours before catheterization. No patient was on amiodarone. No premedication (tranquilizer) was given. Right and left catheterization was performed by the right femoral approach. Catheterization of the coronary sinus was accomplished through the left or right brachial vein. After coronary angiography had been performed and coronary artery disease was excluded, left ventriculography with simultaneous pressure measurement was performed with a 8F Millar microtipped catheter pressure transducer (Houston, Texas). Thereafter, myocardial bloodflow was measured by the argon method; blood samples were taken from the aorta and the coronary sinus for oxygen saturation measurements. Cardiac output was measured by the thermodilution technique.

Hemodynamic measurements

Aortic and left ventricular pressures were measured with pigtail Millar microtipped catheter pressure transducer (PC-485, 8F) in all patients. Left ventriculography was performed at 50 frames/s by power injection of 40 ml nonionic contrast solution. The projection was a $10°$ caudally angulated right anterior oblique view. Left ventricular pressure was recorded

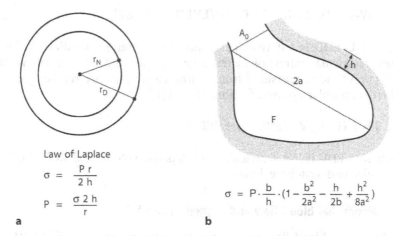

Fig. 1. Formulas of La Place and Mirsky. Using the equation of La Place, the left ventricular chamber is assumed to be a thin-walled sphere (**a**); using the equation of Mirsky, the left ventricular chamber is assumed to be a thick-walled ellipsoid (**b**)

simultaneously. Care was taken to obtain a series of heartbeats without premature left ventricular contractions. Heart rate was determined from the continuous recording of the electrocardiogram. Maximum rate of left ventricular pressure rise was determined from continuous electronic differentiation of left ventricular pressure tracings.

During one cardiac cycle, left ventricular end-diastolic volume was calculated from each cine frame at intervals of 20 ms with the Sandler-Dodge method [27]. Left ventricular muscle mass was calculated by a modification of the method by Rackley et al. [23]. Instantaneous wall thickness was calculated at intervals of 20 ms from wall mass, instantaneous volumes, and major and minor hemiaxis using a special computer program (Herrath II) [31]. Instantaneous midwall stress values were calculated on the basis of the ellipsoid model of Mirsky [19] (Fig. 1).

$$S = P \times b/h \times (1 - b^2/2a^2 - h/2b + h^2/8a^2) \qquad (1)$$

where S is instantaneous wall stress, P is instantaneous left ventricular pressure, h is instantaneous left ventricular wall thickness, a is major hemiaxis, b is minor hemiaxis; a and b were derived from calculated values by the area length method. The systolic stress-time integral (STI, [10^3 dynes s/cm^2]) was calculated by integrating instantaneous stress values from end-diastole to end-systole. Pressure-volume work (PV-work, [mmHg×l]) was analyzed as the area of the pressure volume loop obtained by relating instantaneous pressure to volume every 20 ms. Cardiac output was measured by the thermodilution technique, and stroke volume was obtained by dividing cardiac output by heart rate. Mean velocity of circumferential fiber shortening (MV$_{Cf}$ [circ/s]) was derived from the formula:

$$MV_{Cf} = (LVEDD - LVESD)/(LVEDD \times LVET) \tag{2}$$

where LVEDD is left ventricular minor diameter at end-diastole, LVESD is left ventricular minor diameter at end-systole, and LVET is left ventricular ejection time as measured from central aortic pressure recordings.
Left ventricular ejection fraction (EF [%]) is

$$EF = (LVEDV - LVESV)/LVEDV \tag{3}$$

when LVEDV is left ventricular end-diastolic volume and LVESV is left ventricular end-systolic volume.

Myocardial blood flow and oxygen consumption

Myocardial blood flow was measured by the argon method [13, 24]. Argon blood concentrations were measured by gas chromatography [6]. Myocardial oxygen consumption [ml/min/100 g] was determined as the product of myocardial blood flow multiplied by the artery-coronary-sinus-oxygen-content-difference [ml/100 ml]. The latter was derived from oxygen saturation measurements by oxymetry (AO Unisat Oximeter, Dallas, Texas). Myocardial oxygen consumption per beat [μl/100 g/beat] was calculated from myocardial oxygen consumption per minute and heart rate. External myocardial efficiency was calculated as the ratio between the pressure-volume work normalized for 100 g muscle mass and myocardial oxygen consumption per beat [μl/100 g/beat]. Energy units were converted from mmHg×l into cal assuming 1 mmHg×l = 31.79 mcal and 1 μl O_2 = 5 mcal.

Statistics

The statistical analysis was performed using the SPSS/PC + computer program [20]. Linear regression analysis was used for the relation between myocardial oxygen consumption and hemodynamic variables. Differences between the mean values of the two groups were analyzed by an unpaired t-test. Potential differences between slopes and intercepts of the regression lines were analyzed using the t-test according to Sachs [26]. Multiple regression analysis was also performed for taking into account additional hemodynamic variables [20]. Probability values of less than 0.05 were accepted as being significant.

Muscle experiments

Methods regarding isolated cardiac muscle experiments from human hearts are described in detail elsewhere [14–16].

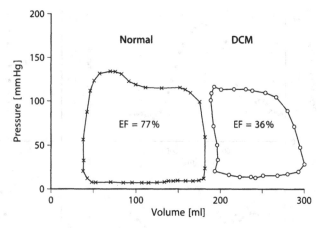

Fig. 2. Pressure-volume relationships of two representative subjects. The respective ejection fractions are also indicated. *DCM:* dilated cardiomyopathy

Table 1. Left ventricular size and function in normal and dilated ventricles

	N	IDC	P
LVEDV [ml]	158±30	343±96	<0.001
LVESV [ml]	56±29	225±102	<0.001
EF [%]	75±7	36±12	<0.001
LVMM [g]	179±37	320±71	<0.001

LVEDV left ventricular end-diastolic volume; *LVESV* left ventricular end-systolic volume; *EF ejection fraction; LVMM* left ventricular muscle mass; *N normal ventricle; IDC idiopathic* dilated cardiomyopathy

■ Results

Left ventricular size, wall mass, and ejection fraction

Chamber dimensions are significantly altered in dilated cardiomyopathy: LVEDV was 159±30 ml in normal and 343±96 ml (p<0.001) in dilated ventricles (Table 1), whereas LVESV was 56±29 ml and 225±102 ml, respectively. Therefore, EF was decreased from 75±7% in normal to 36±12% in dilated ventricles (Table 1; Fig. 2). Left ventricular wall mass was 320±71 g in dilated cardiomyopathy compared to 179±37 in normal ventricles (p<0.001) (Table 1, Fig. 3).

Pressure measurements and hemodynamic variables

There were no significant differences between the groups regarding heart rate, systolic blood pressure, and right atrial pressure (Table 2). Maximum rate of left ventricular pressure rise (dP/dt_{max}) was significantly (p<0.001)

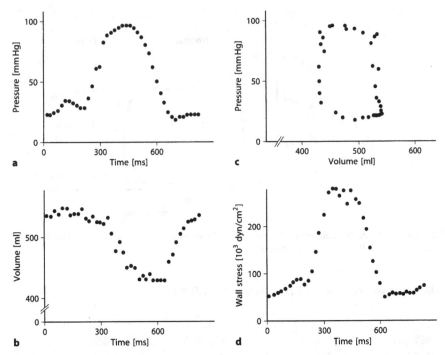

Fig. 3. Quantification of geometrical parameters and stress data in a representative patient with dilated cardiomyopathy. **a** Function between pressure and time. **b** Function between volume and time. **c** Function between pressure and volume. **d** Function between systolic wall stress and time. Data acquisition was obtained every 20 ms; calculation procedure and the computer program have been developed and published by Herrath et al. [31]

decreased from 1509 ± 570 in normal to 1027 ± 262 mmHg/s in dilated ventricles (Table 2). Cardiac output and left ventricular systolic presssure were not significantly different between the groups (Table 2). Pressure-volume work was 11.55 ± 4.96 and 10.41 ± 3.77 mmHg×l in normal and dilated ventricles, respectively (NS, Table 2). Whereas peak systolic wall stress was not significantly different beween the groups, the systolic stress-time integral is increased by 42% (p<0.001) in dilated ventricles (Fig. 5). From representative systolic stress curves in Fig. 4, it can be seen that peak systolic wall stress is reached later and maintained for a longer time, and thereby, relaxation starts later in the dilated ventricles.

Myocardial blood flow and oxygen consumption measurements

Neither myocardial blood flow nor myocardial oxygen consumption per min nor myocardial oxygen consumption per beat were significantly different between the groups (Table 3).

Table 2. Hemodynamic parameters in normal and dilated ventricles

	N	IDC	P
HR [1/min]	80.89 ± 16.07	85.76 ± 15.73	N.S.
SAP [mmHg]	138.74 ± 20.01	127.70 ± 15.99	N.S.
DAP [mmHg]	74.89 ± 8.74	71.95 ± 9.50	N.S.
dP/dt$_{max}$ [mmHg/s]	1509.37 ± 570.33	1026.70 ± 262.37	P<0.01
LVEDP [mmHg]	9.26 ± 4.37	18.00 ± 8.75	P<0.01
CO [l/min]	6.51 ± 1.41	6.01 ± 1.16	N.S.
LVSP [mmHg]	133.81 ± 32.22	117.97 ± 17.50	N.S.
∫P×V [mmHg l]	11.55 ± 4.96	10.41 ± 3.77	N.S.
PSS [10³dyn/cm²]	236.3 ± 57.9	273.0 ± 55.2	N.S.
STI [10³dyn×s/cm²]	76.52 ± 21.06	109.74 ± 26.68	P<0.001
MV$_{CF}$ [circ/s]	1.56 ± 0.42	0.61 ± 0.24	P<0.001

HR Heart rate; *SAP* systolic arterial pressure; *DAP* diastolic arterial pressure; *dP/dt$_{max}$* maximum rise of pressure development; *LVEDP* left ventricular end-diastolic pressure; *CO* cardiac output; *LVSP* left ventricular systolic pressure; *∫P·V* pressure-volume work; *PSS* peak systolic wall stress; *STI* systolic stress-time integral; *MV$_{CF}$* mean circumferential fiber shortening; *N* normal ventricles; *IDC* idiopathic dilated cardiomyopathy.

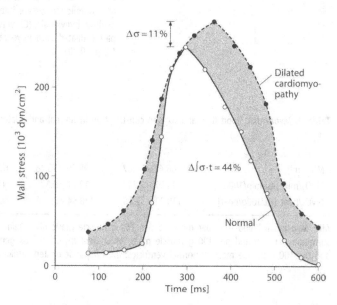

Fig. 4. Representative systolic wall stress curves as a function of time of a normal and a dilated left ventricle. Whereas the difference between systolic stress is small and not of statistical significance, the systolic stress-time integral was 42% greater (p < 0.001) in patients with dilated cardiomyopathy. Mean data see Fig. 5

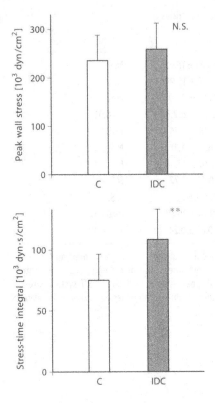

Fig. 5. Peak systolic wall stress (*upper columns*) and systolic stress-time integral (*lower columns*) in healthy individuals (C) versus patients with idiopathic dilated cardiomyopathy (IDC). NS, $p > 0.05$; **, $p < 0.001$

Table 3. Myocardial blood flow and oxygen consumption in normal and dilated ventricles

	N	IDC	P
MBF [ml]	88.42×27.87	95.59×30.26	N.S.
MVO$_2$/min [ml/min/100g]	11.07×2.71	12.07×3.52	N.S.
MVO$_2$/beat [µl/100g/beat]	138.42×32.18	140.54×35.56	N.S.

MBF Myocardial blood flow per min and per 100 g muscle mass; *MVO$_2$/min* myocardial oxygen consumption per min and per 100 g muscle mass; *MVO$_2$/beat* myocardial oxygen consumption per beat and per 100 g muscle mass; *N* normal ventricles; *IDC* idiopathic dilated cardiomyopathy

External efficiency and its relation of left ventricular end-diastolic volume

External efficiency was calculated from pressure-volume work and myocardial oxygen consumption per beat. It was $31 \pm 12\%$ in normal and decreased to $16 \pm 6\%$ in dilated ventricles. In dilated cardiomyopathy, a significant correlation was found for the relation between efficiency and left ven-

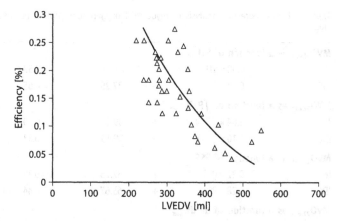

Fig. 6. External efficiency as a function of left ventricular end-diastolic volume. A significant ($p < 0.001$) and inverse correlation was found

tricular end-diastolic volume (Fig. 6; $r = 0.68$; $p < 0.01$). Figure 6 also indicates that in very large left ventricles myocardial efficiency may be as low as 5 to 10%.

Coupling between myocardial oxygen consumption and hemodynamic variables

Linear regression analysis was performed for analyzing the relationship between myocardial oxygen consumption per beat and the following mechanical parameters: systolic stress-time integral, peak systolic wall stress, pressure-volume work, maximum rate of left ventricular pressure rise, and mean velocity of circumferential shortening. In normal ventricles, myocardial oxygen consumption per beat correlated best with the systolic stress-time integral (Table 4; $r = 0.59$; $p < 0.01$), whereas the correlation between myocardial oxygen consumption per beat with mean velocity of circumferential fiber shortening was of less relevance (Table 4; $r = 0.54$; $p < 0.05$). Additionally, this latter function showed a negative and very flat slope (Table 4). For the relation between myocardial oxygen consumption and left ventricular pressure-volume work, peak systolic wall stress or dP/dt_{max}, no significant correlation could be found (Table 4). Using multiple regression analysis, additional consideration of dP/dt_{max} or mean velocity of circumferential fiber shortening did not improve the oxygen consumption versus stress-time integral correlation.

In the group of patients with idiopathic dilated cardiomyopathy, the best correlation was found again between myocardial oxygen consumption per beat and the systolic stress-time integral (Table 4; $r = 0.65$; $p < 0.001$). The correlations between myocardial oxygen consumption per beat and pressure-volume work ($r = 0.33$; $p < 0.05$) or peak systolic wall stress ($r = 0.44$; $p < 0.01$) were of less significance. No significant correlation was found

Table 4. Linear regression analysis of myocardial oxygen consumption per beat and mechanical variables

MVO_{2beat} as a function of STI

N	$0.90 \times STI$	+	69.34	$r = 0.59$	$p < 0.01$
IDC	$0.94 \times STI$	+	37.25	$r = 0.65$	$p < 0.001$

MVO_{2beat} as a function of $\int P \cdot V$

N	$2.64 \times \int P \cdot V$	+	109.34	$r = 0.40$	N.S.
IDC	$3.10 \times \int P \cdot V$	+	109.13	$r = 0.33$	$p < 0.05$

MVO_{2beat} as a function of PSS

N	$0.22 \times PSS$	+	87.75	$r = 0.39$	N.S.
IDC	$0.28 \times PSS$	+	65.67	$r = 0.44$	$p < 0.01$

MVO_{2beat} as a function of dP/dt_{max}

N	$-0.0003 \times dP/dt_{max}$	+	138.92	$r = 0.01$	N.S.
IDC	$0.014 \times dP/dt_{max}$	+	125.97	$r = 0.11$	N.S.

MVO_{2beat} as a function of MV_{CF}

N	$-41.36 \times MV_{CF}$	+	203.08	$r = 0.54$	$p < 0.05$
IDC	$8.70 \times MV_{CF}$	+	135.22	$r = 0.06$	N.S.

MVO_{2beat} myocardial oxygen consumption per beat; *STI* systolic stress-time integral; $\int P \cdot V$ pressure-volume work; *PSS* peak systolic stress; dP/dt_{max} maximum rise of pressure development; MV_{CF} mean velocity of circumferential fiber shortening; *N* normal ventricles; *IDC* idiopathic dilated cardiomyopathy

between myocardial oxygen consumption per beat and dP/dt_{max} or mean velocity of fiber shortening (Table 4). Using multiple regression analysis, the correlation between myocardial oxygen consumption per beat and stress-time integral could not be improved by taking into account additional parameters. Therefore, the systolic stress-time integral which reflects best myocardial energy demand is increased by 42% in dilated ventricles.

■ Discussion

Patients population

In the present study, individuals with normal cardiac function and dimensions were compared to patients with idiopathic dilated cardiomyopathy. These patients showed moderately to severely enlarged ventricles; those with moderate dilative cardiomyopathy had ventricles which were only slighly greater than 220 ml at end-diastole. On the other hand, the most severely ill patients had ventricles with enddiastolic volumes more than 400 ml. Therefore, a whole range of enlarged left ventricles was studied. In this context it is important to realize that all of the patients were well compensated. In a decompensated state, left ventricular volumes of each patient may be greater. This means that the geometrical and mechanical parameters measured in our patients are measured in the best clinical situations indicating that these parameters are poor at the beginning of decompensation and are worst at full decompensation.

Average differences between normal and enlarged ventricles are evident. End-diastolic volumes are doubled, ejection fraction is halved, left ventricular end-diastolic pressure is doubled, and dP/dt_{max} as well as circumferential fiber shortening, two parameters of LV contractility, are severely decreased.

Stress-time integral and MVO$_2$

The major determinants of myocardial oxygen consumption that have been postulated so far are heart rate, systolic wall stress or stress-time integral and velocity of myocardial contraction, whereas the relevance of left ventricular pressure volume work is less clear [5, 8, 29, 32].

Since the mechanical parameters are obtained from one cardiac cycle, heart rate was considered by calculating myocardial oxygen consumption per beat. This implies that the ratio between myocardial oxygen consumption per beat and mechanical variables is not substantially influenced by changes in heart rate per se. Accordingly, Rooke and Feigl [25] demonstrated that myocardial oxygen consumption per beat is not substantially influenced by heart rate when hemodynamic variables were kept constant.

In normal and in dilated ventricles, the best correlation was found for the function between myocardial oxygen consumption per beat and systolic stress-time integral. The correlation coefficient was higher in dilated ventricles ($p < 0.01$; $r = 0.59$). In both groups, other parameters were less relevant, and the function of myocardial oxygen consumption versus stress-time integral could not be significantly improved by taking into account other parameters using multiple regression analysis. The systolic stress-time integral describes the pattern of stress development and maintenance thereby reflecting the entire period of mechanical activity [1, 17] (see Fig. 4). This explains why systolic stress-time integral is *the* determinant of myocardial oxygen consumption – both in normal and dilated ventricles.

External efficiency in normal and dilated ventricles

External efficiency is defined as pressure-volume work divided by myocardial oxygen consumption per beat, both normalized for 100 g muscle tissue. This efficiency was calculated to be 31% on the average in the normal hearts. This is more than the originally reported value of 23% [4]. The difference may be due to the different methods used for quantification of left ventricular work. On the other hand, the present data are in good agreement with those of Baxley et al. [7] who reported values as high as 30% for some patients with pressure or volume overload and values as low as 10% for dilated ventricles. In our patients, the lowest efficiency analyzed was around 10%. It is of clinical importance that external myocardial efficiency is closely and inversely related to left ventricular end-diastolic volume. Left ventricular dilatation per se implicates less efficient working conditions so that the myocardium needs more energy for activation processes and force generation than for work performance. Furthermore, this data indicates that an important goal of long-term therapy is due to decrease chamber size in order to keep myocardial efficiency high (see Fig. 3).

Increased stress-time integral versus decreased myocardial efficiency

Despite the development of cardiac hypertrophy, i.e., an increase in left ventricular muscle mass by 84% (compared to normal), myocardial stress can not be compensated. Although peak developed systolic stress is only slightly and nonsignificantly increased in dilated ventricles, the systolic stress-time integral is increased by 42% indicating enhanced afterload during the whole ejection period (Fig. 4).

In order to figure out in what way a 42% increase in afterload may alter stroke volume, work, and efficiency, additional experiments were conducted in isolated preparations from human left ventricular myocardium. These preparations were allowed to contract isotonically against constant afterload (see Fig. 7). When force and extent of shortening are measured, myocardial work can be calculated and plotted as a function of developed force. A typical bell-shaped curve is obtained (Fig. 7) indicating the highest work is reached at medium force, i.e., medium afterload or stress-time integral. In contrast to the experimental situation where the afterload is constant during one cardiac cycle, the in vivo contraction is negative-auxotonic, i.e., systolic stress rapidly decreases during the ejection period because left ventricular size decreases and shorter long axis and short axis radii allow low stress at constant intraventricular pressure (Fig. 1). Therefore, integrated systolic stress over time, i.e., stress-time integral, needs to be taken into account. If the clinically obtained stress-time integral data are incorporated into the experimental data (Fig. 8), it can be seen that an increase in stress-time integral necessarily leads to a decrease in work. This implies also a decease in stroke volume and myocardial efficiency. In numbers it means that an increase in systolic stress-time integral of 42% is followed by a 30% reduction in work or stroke volume. As a consequence, heart and circulation react by neuroendocrine activation in order to compensate for low stroke volume. However, in heart failure these mechanisms may not act properly because of down-regulation of β-adrenoceptors [7] and a reversed force-frequency relation [12].

As a therapeutic strategy, it may be a smart goal to keep left ventricular dimensions small! This may be reached controversally by application of vasodilators and diuretics or – at later stages of heart failure – by surgical reverse remodeling of the left ventricle [2, 9, 30]. From a pathophysiological point of view, both methods might work by optimizing geometrical factors thereby reducing systolic stress-time integral and increasing stroke volume, work, and myocardial efficiency.

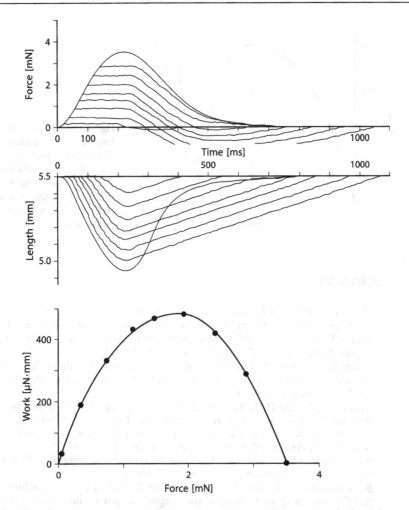

Fig. 7. Typical records of force development (*upper panel*) and shortening (*middle panel*) obtained in a left ventricular human muscle preparation contracting against a variety of afterloads. When multiplying the afterload (force) by the respective extent of shortening (length), the external work performed by the muscle is obtained for each contraction. Plotting the calculated work as a function of the corresponding afterload the typical well-shaped work-load relation is obtained (*lower panel*). Note that maximum work is performed at medium afterload. Muscle length 5.5 mm, experimental temperature 37 °C, stimulation rate 30 per min

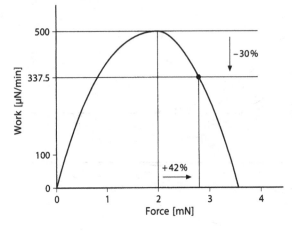

Fig. 8. Work as a function of force (constant afterload); same well-shaped curve as in lower panel of Fig. 7. A 42% increase of afterload – as analyzed for the stress-time integral in patients – leads to a 30% reduction of myocardial work

▪ References

1. Alpert NR, Mulieri LA, Litten RZ (1983) Isoenzyme contribution to economy of contraction and relaxation in normal and hypertrophied hearts. In: Jacob R, Guelch W, Kissling G (eds) Cardiac Adaption to Hemodynamic Overload, Training and Stress. Darmstadt, Steinkopf Verlag, pp 147–157
2. Batista RJV, Santos JLV, Takeshita N, Bocchino L, Lima PN, Cunha MA (1996) Partial left ventriculectomy to improve left ventricular function in end-stage heart disease. J Card Surg II:96–97
3. Baxley WA, Dodge HAT, Rackley CE, Sandler H, Pugh D (1977) Left ventricular mechanical efficiency in man with heart disease. Circulation 55:564–568
4. Bing RJ, Hammond MM, Handelsman JC, Powers SR, Spencer FC, Eckenhoff JE, Goodale WT, Haffens HJ, Kety SS (1949) Am Heart J 38:1–24
5. Braunwald E (1971) Control of myocardial oxygen consumption. Physiological and clinical considerations. Am J Cardiol 27:416–432
6. Bretschneider HJ, Cott L, Hilgert G, Probst R, Rau G (1966) Gaschromatographische Trennung und Analyse von Argon als Basis einer neuen Fremdgasmethode zur Durchblutungsmessung von Organen. Verh Dtsch Ges Kreisl-Forsch 32:267–273
7. Brodde OE (1991) β_1- and β_2-adrenoceptors in the human heart: properties, function, and alterations in chronic heart failure. Pharmacol Rev 43:203–242
8. Coleman HN, Sonnenblick EH, Braunwald E (1969) Myocardial oxygen consumption associated with external work: The Fenn effect. Am J Physiol 217:291–296
9. Frazier OH, Radovancevic B, Odegaard P, Hernandez A, Wilansky S, Cook P (1997) Left ventricular reduction in patients with idiopathic cardiomyopathy awaiting heart transplantation – preliminary results. J Heart Lung Transplant 16:80
10. Gillbert EM, Abraham WT, Olsen S, Hattler B, White M, Mealy P, Larrabee P, Bristow MR (1996) Comparative hemodynamic, left ventricular functional, and beta-adrenergic effects of chronic treatment with metoprolol versus carvedilol in the failing heart. Circulation 94:2817–2825
11. Grossmann W (1986) Profiles in valvular heart disease. In: Grossmann W (ed): Cardiac Catheterization and Angiography. Philadelphia, Lea & Febinger, pp 359–381

12. Hasenfuss G, Reinecke H, Studer R, Holubarsch Ch, Just H, Drexler H (1994) Relation between myocardial function and expression of sarcoplasmic Ca^{2+}-ATPase in failing and nonfailing human myocardium. Circ Res 75:4334–4343
13. Heiss HW, Blümchen G (1982) Durchblutungsmessungen am Koronargefäßsystem. In: Reindell H, Roskamm H (eds): Herzkrankheiten. Heidelberg/New York, Springer Verlag, Inc, pp 413–422
14. Holubarsch Ch, Hasenfuss G, Schmidt-Schweda S, Knorr A, Pieske B, Ruf T, Fasol R, Just H (1993) Angiotensin I and II exert inotropic effects in atrial but not in ventricular myocardium. Circulation 88:1228–1237
15. Holubarsch Ch, Lüdemann J, Wiesner S, Ruf T, Schulte-Baukloh H, Schmidt-Schweda S, Pieske B, Posival H, Just H (1998) Shortening versus isometric contractions in isolated human failing and non-failing left ventricular myocardium: dependency of external work and force on muscle length, heart rate and inotropic stimulation. Cardiovascular Research 37:46–57
16. Holubarsch Ch, Ruf T, Goldstein DJ, Ashton RC, Nickl W, Pieske B, Pioch K, Lüdemann J, Wiesner S, Hasenfuss G, Posival H, Just H, Burkhoff D (1996) Existence of the Frank-Starling mechanism in the failing human heart. Investigations on the organ, tissue, and sarcomere levels. Circulation 94:683–689
17. Laskey WK, Reichek N, Sutton MS, Untereker WJ, Hirshfeld JW (1983) Myocardial oxygen consumption in left ventricular hypertrophy and its relation to left ventricular mechanics. Am J Cardiol 52:852–858
18. McCarthy PM, Starling RC, Smedira NG, Buda TM, Scaha GM, Young JB (1997) Partial ventriculectomy with valve repair as an alternative to cardiac transplantation. J Heart Lung Transplant 16:41
19. Mirsky I (1979) Elastic properties of the myocardium: A quatitative approach with physiological and clinical application. In: Berne RM (ed) Handbook of Physiology. The Cardiovascular System. Washington, DC, American Physiological Society, pp 497–531
20. Norusis MJ (1986) SPSS/PC+. Chicago, SPSS Inc.
21. Packer M, Bristow MR, Cohn JN, Colucci WS, Fowler MB, Gilbert EM, Shusterman NH (1996) The effect of carvedilol on morbidity and mortality in patients with chronic heart failure. N Engl J Med 334:1348–1355
22. Pfeffer MA, Braunwald, E, Moge LA et al. for the SAVE investigators (1992) Effect of captopril on mortality and morbidity in patients with left ventricular dysfunction and myocardial infarction. N Engl J Med 327:669–677
23. Rackley CE, Dodge HT, Coble YD, Hay RE (1964) A method for determining left ventricular mass in man. Circulation 29:666–671
24. Rau G (1969) Messung der Koronardurchblutung mit der Argon-Fremdgasmethode. Arch Kreisl-Forschung 58:322–398
25. Rooke GA, Feigl EO (1982) Work as correlate of canine left ventricular oxygen consumption, and the problem of catecholamine oxygen wasting. Circ Res 50:273–286
26. Sachs L (1984) Angewandte Statistik. 6. Auflage. Springer Verlag Berlin, Heidelberg, New York, Tokyo
27. Sandler H, Dodge HT, Coble YD, Hay RE (1968) The use of single plane angiocardiograms for the calculation of the left ventricular volume in man. Am Heart J 75:325–334
28. The SOLVD Investigators (1991) Effects of enalapril on survival in patients with reduced left ventricular ejection fraction and congestive heart failure. N Engl J Med 325:293–302
29. Strauer B (1979) Ventricular function and coronary hemodynamics in hypertensive heart disease. Am J Cardiol 44:999–1006

30. Takeshita N, Kawaguchi AT, Lima RRN, Bocchino L, Verde LJ, Batista JVR (1997) Hemodynamic changes in patients undergoing left ventricular diameter reduction (Batista operation). J Am Coll Cardiol 29:64A
31. v. Herrath M, Holubarsch Ch, Hasenfuss G, Heiss HW, Just H (1990) Repeat determination of left ventricular wall thickness from mass and volume during one cardiac cycle. Clinical Cardiology 13:218–220
32. Weber KT, Janicki JS (1977) Myocardial oxygen consumption. The role of wall force and shortening. Am J Physiol 233:H421–H430

Author's address:

Prof. Dr. Ch. J. F. Holubarsch
Department of Cardiology and Angiology
Medizinische Universitätsklinik Freiburg
Hugstetter Strasse 55
D-79106 Freiburg, Germany
E-mail: holubarsch@mm31.ukl.uni-freiburg.de

CHAPTER **8** # Mitral valve repair for surgical remodeling

S. F. BOLLING and I. A. SMOLENS

■ Background

Congestive heart failure is one of the leading causes of hospitalization in the United States today and its incidence in the population is increasing. Heart failure will become even more of a medical challenge as average life expectancy continues to rise. Despite significant improvements with medical management; approximately 50% of patients with congestive heart failure die within three years of clinical presentation [63]. While heart transplantation is now considered standard treatment for select patients with severe congestive heart failure, it is only applicable to a small percentage of these patients. Transplantation is limited both by the small number of donor hearts available and its inapplicability in the older patient or those with comorbid medical conditions that would preclude them from consideration [37]. In the effort to address this problem, alternative and new surgical strategies have evolved including coronary artery revascularization [24, 25], mechanical circulatory support [28, 31, 52], cardiomyoplasty [45, 48], left ventricular myoreduction [7, 8], and mitral valve repair [5, 6, 15, 16, 21].

Many patients with cardiomyopathy develop significant mitral regurgitation. Historically, the surgical approach to patients with mitral regurgitation was mitral valve replacement and little was understood about the adverse consequences that interruption of the annulus-papillary muscle continuity had on left ventricular systolic function [55]. This procedure was associated with very high mortality rates [53, 54]. It is in this population of patients that the concept of the "pop off" effect of mitral regurgitation originated, that is, reversal of blood flow was somehow beneficial to the patient in heart failure. It has been demonstrated in a number of studies that preservation of the annulus-papillary muscle continuity is of paramount importance to preservation of left ventricular function [22, 59]. It was the excision of and disruption of the subvalvar apparatus that accounted for the significant loss of systolic function due to the destruction of the left ventricle that led to the poor outcome in patients who underwent mitral valve replacement [36, 60]. Preservation of the mitral valve apparatus and left ventricle in mitral valve repair has been demonstrated to enhance and maintain left ventricular function and geometry with an associated decrease in wall stress [30, 64]. This procedure has been shown to be safe with a significant decrease in operative morbidity and mortality with good long-term outcomes [2, 3, 29, 56]. In fact, it has been shown that there is no "pop-off" effect but the mortality ascribed to these patients from mitral valve repair was due to the disruption of the subvalvar apparatus and loss of left ventricular function.

■ Mitral valve repair

At the University of Michigan between June 1993 and January 1999, 92 patients with end-stage cardiomyopathy and refractory severe mitral regurgitation were studied prospectively. All patients had NYHA Class III or IV congestive heart failure despite receiving maximal medical therapy (digoxin, diuretics, and afterload reducing agents), and had severe left ventricular systolic dysfunction as defined by an ejection fraction <25% on angiography or radionuclide studies. Patient ages ranged from 33 to 81 years (mean 60 ± 5 years). Patients were equally divided between nonischemic dilated cardiomyopathy and end-stage ischemic cardiomyopathy without ongoing ischemia, as defined by a negative dobutamine echocardiogram and or a negative positron emission tomography scan. No patient was believed to have any ongoing ischemia and would therefore not be expected to gain any improvement from a coronary artery revascularization procedure. The mean duration of documented cardiomyopathy or symptomatic heart failure was 3 ± 6 years (range 0–16 years). Preoperative ejection fraction ranged from 8 to 24% (mean 14%). At surgery all patients underwent mitral valve reconstruction with implantation of an undersized flexible annuloplasty remodeling ring, no patient underwent a complex mitral valve repair. Mitral valve reconstruction was performed via median sternotomy with cardiopulmonary bypass, utilizing hypothermic, blood cardioplegic arrest in primary patients and via right thoracotomy, utilizing cold fibrillatory arrest in 38 redo patients who had undergone prior coronary artery bypass grafting.

There was one intra-operative mortality from right ventricular failure in a patient who despite both the use of the intra-aortic balloon pump (IABP) and mechanical right ventricular assist device support was unable to survive. Five patients required IABP support, and there were no patients who required the use of a left ventricular assist device. Intra-operative transesophageal echocardiography revealed no mitral regurgitation in most patients and mild regurgitation in 7. All patients were weaned from cardiopulmonary bypass and maintained in the immediate post-operative period on milrinone (a phosphodiesterase inhibitor) and norepinephrine infusions. The overall operative mortality was 5%. There were five 30-day mortalities: one due to cardiac failure, one due to a stroke, two due to multisystem organ failure, primarily related to underlying pulmonary failure, and the one intraoperative death mentioned previously.

The duration of follow-up in these patients has been 1–68 months (mean 38 months), with a one and two year actuarial survival of 80% and

Table 1. Preoperative and postoperative echocardiographic data

ECHO parameter	Preoperative	Postoperative (24 month)	P Value
End diastolic volume (ml)	281 ± 86	206 ± 88	< 0.001
Ejection fraction (%)	16 ± 5	26 ± 8	0.008
Regurgitant fraction (%)	70 ± 12	13 ± 10	< 0.001
Cardiac output (L/min)	3.1 ± 1.0	5.2 ± 0.8	0.001
Sphericity index (D/L)	0.82 ± 0.10	0.74 ± 0.07	0.005

70%, respectively. All patients remain on medical therapy for their congestive heart failure. On immediate post-operative echocardiograms, the mean trans-mitral gradient was 3 ± 1 mmHg (range 2–6 mmHg); there were no cases of mitral stenosis or systolic anterior motion (SAM). At 24-month follow-up, all remaining patients are in NYHA Class I or II, with a mean ejection fraction of 26% and with a demonstrated improvement in ejection fraction in each patient and in the group as a whole. A marked reduction in regurgitant volume and regurgitant fraction was demonstrated. The NYHA Class improved for each patient individually and from a mean of 3.2 ± 0.2 to 1.8 ± 0.4 for the entire group. All patients reported subjective improvement in functional status. In those patients whom preoperative data was available for comparison, peak maximal volume of O_2 use during a six minute walk rose significantly from a mean of 14.5 to 18.6 ml O_2/kg/min. Follow-up data for all patients are available at 24 months. The matched preoperative and 24 month postoperative echocardiographic data are recorded in Table 1. All patients had a reduction in sphericity index and regurgitant fraction. All patients demonstrated improvement in left ventricular ejection fraction, cardiac output, and end diastolic volumes. There have been 26 late deaths. This number includes three patients who had further progression of disease and have undergone transplantation and two deaths were related to complications following other operative procedures. The other deaths have resulted from progression of heart failure (n = 8), despite no significant return of mitral regurgitation, sudden ventricular arrhythmia (n=12, 8 in ischemic patients), and one suicide.

■ Pathophysiology

In order to address the issue of heart failure and mitral regurgitation, one needs to first understand the anatomy of the mitral valve. The determination of mitral competence depends on the understanding that the mitral valve apparatus consists of the annulus, leaflets, chordae tendinae, papillary muscles, and the entire left ventricle. Maintenance of the chordal, annular, subvalvar continuity, and mitral geometric relationships are important in the preservation of overall ventricular function and may be even more important in patients with compromised left ventricular function. In the selection of a surgical approach to the problem of heart failure, one must therefore first recognize that this is a ventricular problem and therefore a solution directed at the mitral valve, which is and encompasses the entire left ventricle, would be ideal. Excision of a portion of the left ventricular wall does not address the issue directly and in fact can further disrupt the mitral valve apparatus by disruption of the left ventricular wall.

Functional mitral regurgitation is a significant complication of end stage cardiomyopathy and may effect almost all heart failure patients as a preterminal or terminal event. The mitral regurgitation develops secondary to an alteration in the annular-ventricular apparatus [17] and altered ventricular geometry [43], which results in incomplete leaflet coaptation. In ischemic cardiomyopathy this can be attributed to papillary or lateral wall muscle dysfunction, and in nonischemic cardiomyopathy it is ascribed to annular dilation and chordal tethering [38]. The mitral regurgitation exacerbates the volume overload [69] of the already dilated ventricle with further progression of annular dilation, increased left ventricular wall tension, worsening mitral regurgitation, and increased failure, which is predictive of a poor outcome [10].

For patients with dilated cardiomyopathy, mortality is directly related to severity of ventricular systolic dysfunction [10]. In addition, increased chamber sphericity and, more importantly, the presence of mitral insufficiency [39] are markers of a worse prognosis. In review of these types of patients, 1-year mortality has been reported between 54% and 70% [4, 39]. Furthermore, in a study of 28 patients awaiting transplantation, with an ejection fraction of 25% or less, 1-year survival was only 46% and independent predictors of death were low forward stroke volumes, history of ventricular arrhythmias, and mitral regurgitation [61].

■ Relationship to orifice area

The pathogenesis of the myopathy related mitral regurgitation is multifactorial. In the absence of organic disease, mitral regurgitation is predominantly thought to occur as a result of progressive dilation of the mitral annulus with subsequent loss of coaptation of the valve leaflets. A large leaflet area is normally required for coaptation because mitral leaflet area is 2½; times greater than the area of the mitral valve orifice. As more mitral leaflet tissue is utilized for coverage of the enlarging mitral valve orifice, a critical reduction in the leaflet tissue available for coaptation is reached, such that coaptation of the mitral valve leaflets becomes ineffective, and a central regurgitant jet of "functional" insufficiency begins to develop [17, 20]. Therefore, the most significant determinants of mitral valve coaptation, leaflet orifice area, and mitral regurgitation are the dimensions of the mitral valve annulus. The left ventricular dimension is a less important factor in functional mitral regurgitation, because chordal length and papillary muscle length are not significantly different in people with idiopathic cardiomyopathy with or without mitral regurgitation [17].

In ischemic cardiomyopathy, the mechanisms that contribute to mitral regurgitation are complex. They may include "functional" mitral regurgitation, through dilation of the mitral valve annulus, and "papillary muscle dysfunction", which is an unsuccessful coordination of the entire mitral valve apparatus rather than simply an isolated disorder of the papillary muscle [40]. These ischemic related changes are again all thought to result in an insufficient area of coaptation of the mitral leaflets.

In a recent study of patients with severe heart failure, who were managed with pharmacologic agents (diuretics, nitrates, and afterload reduction agents), the observed decrease in filling pressure and systemic vascular resistance led to a reduction in the dynamic mitral regurgitation associated with their heart failure. This was attributed to a reduction in the regurgitant orifice area related to the decrease in left ventricular volume and annular distension [57]. This complex relationship between mitral annular area and leaflet coaptation may explain why, paradoxically, an undersized "valvular" repair can help a "muscular" problem. Although significant undersizing of the mitral annulus was employed in our study to over correct for the zone of coaptation, no mitral stenosis was induced nor was any SAM noted. SAM was avoided due to widening of the aorto-mitral angle and increased left ventricular size seen in myopathic patients. In addition, acute remodeling of the base of the heart from the undersizing of the mitral annular ring may also contribute to the improvement seen in these myopathic hearts. This may reestablish the ellipsoid shape and somewhat normal geometry to the base of the left ventricle.

■ Ventricular adaptations

Increases in left ventricular preload, wall tension, diastolic volume, and stroke volume are all documented ventricular adaptations to severe mitral regurgitation. There is a significant decrease in the efficiency of the left ventricular contraction and the work expended by the left ventricle to produce flow that ultimately does not contribute to effective forward cardiac output. In these patients, maintenance of forward flow becomes more difficult because up to 50% of the stroke volume is ejected into the left atrium before the aortic valve even opens [25]. With elimination of the regurgitant volume, the ventricle no longer has to expend an excessive amount of work on flow that is going in the reverse direction. All blood flow will be in the forward direction, and will contribute to forward flow and effective cardiac output. In cases of severe myocardial dysfunction, the positive effects of the elimination of the regurgitant flow may be even more pronounced.

▪ Coronary flow characteristics

Further evidence of underlying mechanisms why mitral valve repair for patients with cardiomyopathy may be successful is taken from a study of the coronary flow characteristics in patients with mitral regurgitation, in the absence of coronary artery disease. This study assessed coronary flow characteristics in patients before and after mitral valve reconstruction. Coronary flow reserve was limited in patients with mitral regurgitation due to an increase in baseline coronary flow and flow velocity which was related to left ventricular volume overload, hypertrophy, and preload (left ventricular wall stress). The restriction in coronary flow reserve improved following mitral valve reconstruction because of a reduction in the baseline coronary flow and flow velocity once the left ventricular preload, work, and mass were reduced [1]. Based on this study, in patients with mitral regurgitation and cardiomyopathy, a restriction in the coronary flow reserve would seem probable and an improvement in flow reserve and velocity would be expected following mitral valve repair. Ultimately the mitral valve repair in this setting would lead to an improvement in the left ventricular geometry.

▪ Neurohumoral alterations

In the setting of chronic congestive heart failure, when cardiac reserve is depressed, various mechanisms compensate for the reduction in cardiac performance to maintain cardiovascular homeostasis. Some of the well-recognized compensatory mechanisms include an increase in sympathetic nervous system activity with an increase in release of several neurohumoral factors. In response to the increased sympathetic activity, norepinephrine is released from the myocyte into the synaptic cleft and it binds to the β-adrenoceptors. These receptors then couple with adenylyl cyclase, which results in an increase in cyclic AMP (cAMP) production. This leads to the stimulation of protein kinase A and ultimately results in a positive inotropic response [41]. In heart failure there is an excessive release of norepinephrine from the myocardium, a corresponding increase in plasma norepinephrine levels, and a reduction in myocardial stores of norepinephrine [12]. Following long-term exposure to elevated levels of norepinephrine, the numbers of β-adrenoceptors become downregulated [18, 19], the receptors become desensitized, and the post-receptor signal transducing pathway becomes altered [34]. This results in a decrease in cAMP production and a reduced positive inotropic effect of β-adrenoceptor agonists [34, 65]. In addition, while in the setting of heart failure, the positive inotropic effects of phosphodiesterase inhibitors, when used as a single agent, are reduced in comparison to that of the nonfailing heart [12, 13] due to diminished basal cAMP production in the failing heart [14]. It would therefore seem that the administration of β-adrenoceptor agonists or cAMP phosphodiesterase inhibitors would not be the best treatment in patients with heart failure. Additionally, the use of β-adrenoceptor agonists in the acute setting are associated with a high incidence of arrhythmias. In our study population we advocate the simultaneous use of norepinephrine and milrinone. The exogenous norepinephrine administration acts to replete the diminished myocardial stores of norepinephrine and it stimulates cAMP production which has been shown to restore the positive inotropic effects of phosphodiesterase inhibitors [14, 26].

▪ Cytokine response

Heart failure is a clinical syndrome derived from chronic work overload of the myocardium, ischemia, inflammation, and additional etiologies such as cardiomyopathy. Studies have shown that the proinflammatory cytokines tumor necrosis factor-a (TNF-a), IL-1, IL-2, and IL-6 may be responsible for the myocardial depression seen in the complex syndrome of heart failure [11, 44, 51, 66]. TNF-a has been shown to be produced by the heart under stress and has negative inotropic effects. Studies have demonstrated that this proinflammatory cytokine may play a role in the development of left ventricular dysfunction, dilated cardiomyopathy, hypotension, and pulmonary edema, all of which can be manifestations of advanced heart failure [33, 35, 47, 62]. There are two forms of TNF-a specific receptors: TNF-R1 and TNF-R2. Both receptors are found in equal proportions in the normal myocardium and TNF-a binds with equal affinity to both receptors. The negative inotropic effects of TNF-a are mediated primarily by its interaction with TNF-R1. The expression of the myocardial TNF-Rs is downregulated in the presence of heart failure, similar to that seen with the β-adrenergic receptors [35, 67]. The circulating, or soluble, forms of the TNF-Rs are elevated in patients with heart failure suggesting that these receptors may be "shed" from the myocardial cells [27]. The circulating TNF-Rs can neutralize the biological effects of circulating TNF-a [68]. Based on these observations, it has been postulated the cardiac tissue response to increased TNF-a levels is to increase the level of soluble TNF receptors in order to decrease the amount of bioactive TNF-a that can potentially stimulate cardiac cells [35]. At the University of Michigan we have

Table 2. Preoperative and postoperative cytokine levels

	TNF-a (pg/ml)	TNF-R1 (pg/ml)	TNF-R2 (pg/ml)	IL-6 (pg/ml)	IL6-R (ng/ml)
Pre-op	3.5 ± 1.3	931 ± 187	1989 ± 381	61 ± 6.6	36.0 ± 5.2
Post-op (6 mo.)	2.8 ± 1.1	774 ± 177	1450 ± 254	2.9 ± 1.8	31.2 ± 8.1
P value	0.02	<0.01	<0.01	0.13	0.15

measured levels of TNF-a, soluble TNF-R1 and TNF-R2, IL-6 and IL-6 receptors in the pre and post-operative period in patients undergoing mitral valve repair in the presence of heart failure; these data are recorded in Table 2. Six months following mitral reconstruction, the levels of these cytokines and their respective soluble receptor levels were decreased. While this data supports the role of TNF-a in the development of heart failure, further studies are being conducted in which the soluble recombinant form of TNF-R is being administered to heart failure patients in the hope of decreasing some of the manifestations of failure [35].

■ Comparison of left ventricular myoreduction and mitral valve repair

As the availability of transplantation as treatment for patients with end-stage cardiomyopathy is limited, there has been recent interest in the altered geometry of the left ventricle in patients with severe dysfunction. This innovative work was initially described by Batista, who states that all mammalian hearts share the same ratio of mass to diameter, regardless of the size of the heart. The formula that is common to all hearts is muscle mass equals four times the radius cubed ($M = 4 \times R^3$). Batista proposed that for those hearts that do not comply with this relationship they should undergo an operative procedure to restore the ratio back to normal [7, 8]. Surgeons have attempted to renormalize this relationship by left ventricular myoreduction surgery, also called partial left ventricular reduction surgery, reduction myoplasty or the Batista procedure. Batista initially reported an operative mortality of 5%, a 30-day mortality of 22%, and a two-year survival of 55%. Unfortunately, complete and long-term follow-up was not available for these patients [7, 9, 32, 58]. This procedure has met with varying degrees of success in the United States and worldwide [23, 42, 46, 49, 58]. The Cleveland Clinic series of 62 patients (95% idiopathic cardiomyopathy) reported a 3.5% hospital mortality with 7 late deaths and with a one-year actuarial survival of 82% [46]. Of significance, is that in all of these cases a mitral valve repair or replacement occurred routinely as part of the myoreduction procedure. It is therefore very difficult to discern what the exact role of the correction of mitral regurgitation plays in the overall success of the myoreduction procedure. In patients undergoing mitral valve reconstruction alone for myopathy, there is also a re-establishment of a more normal left ventricular mass to volume ratio without the loss of myocardial mass [15, 16]. The average left ventricular volume at 24 month follow-up in our study was over 200 ml, still quite large, while with the left ventricular myoreduction procedure Batista has demonstrated acute reduction of LV volumes to approximately 90–100 ml at the time of operation [32]. There is no loss of ventricular mass with the mitral valve reconstruction alone; however, an appropriate mass/volume ratio is restored. Importantly, there is an acceptable surgical mortality both at 30 days and 1 year for mitral valve reconstruction, which is equivalent to or lower than what has been reported for left ventricular myoreduction procedures [9, 23, 32, 42, 46, 49, 58].

Finally, with the Batista procedure, one must differentiate the effect of abolishment of mitral regurgitation alone versus the addition of the myoreduction. In a study utilizing a dog model, following correction of mitral regurgitation alone, it was demonstrated that the left ventricular remodeling may be rapid and complete with resultant regurgitant fractions of less than 30% [50]. In the University of Michigan study, a decrease in sphericity index and left ventricular volume measurements were demonstrated post-operatively and it is in these patients that the negative cycle of congestive heart failure is interrupted and the surgical unloading of the left ventricle is achieved. These patients may be undergoing a slow self-remodeling from the alteration of the angulation of the base of the heart, stabilization of the mitral annulus or left ventricular unloading all that contribute to a more favorable left ventricular geometry. This tends to occur more frequently in the patients with idiopathic as opposed to those with ischemic cardiomyopathy. In the hearts with end-stage ischemic cardiomyopathy, the potential for remodeling may be limited due to the presence of scar in the ventricular wall.

▪ Summary

In conclusion, mitral reconstruction via an annuloplasty ring effectively corrects mitral regurgitation in cardiomyopathy patients and is a safe procedure in a high-risk population with an acceptable operative mortality rate. Not only has survival in these patients improved but also functional status has changed remarkably. The effects of this procedure in patients with severe myocardial dysfunction may be attributed to a decrease in the regurgitant orifice area, improvement in the efficiency of each contraction with better effective forward flow, an increase in coronary flow reserve, and reversal of some the alterations in the neurohormonal changes seen in heart failure. These changes all contribute to restoration of the normal left ventricular geometric relationship. While longer-term follow-up is necessary with a greater number of patients, we are encouraged by these results and feel that mitral reconstruction offers a new strategy for end-stage cardiomyopathy.

▪ References

1. Akasaka T, Yoshida K, Hozumi T, Takagi T, Kaji S, Kawamoto T, Ueda Y, Okada Y, Morioka S, Yoshikawa J (1998) Restricted coronary flow reserve in patients with mitral regurgitation improves after mitral reconstructive surgery. J Am Coll Cardiol 32:1923–1930
2. Akins CW, Hilgenberg AD, Buckley MJ, Vlahakes GJ, Torchiana DF, Daggett WM, Austen WG (194) Mitral valve reconstruction versus replacement for degenerative or ischemic mitral regurgitation. Ann Thorac Surg 58:668–676

3. Alvarez JM, Deal CW, Loveridge K, Brennan P, Eisenberg R, Ward M, Bhattacharya K, Atkinson SJ, Choong C (1996) Repairing the degenerative mitral valve: ten to fifteen year follow-up. J Thorac Cardiovasc Surg 112:238–247

4. Anguita M, Arizon JM, Bueno G, Latre JM, Sancho M, Torres F, Gimenez D, Concha M, Valles F (1993) Clinical and hemodynamic predictors of survival in patients aged <65 years with severe congestive heart failure secondary to ischemic or nonischemic dilated cardiomyopathy. Am J Cardiol 72(5):413–417

5. Bach DS, Bolling SF (1996) Improvement following correction of secondary mitral regurgitation in end-stage cardiomyopathy with mitral annuloplasty. Am J Cardiol 78:966–969

6. Bach DS, Bolling SF (1995) Early improvement in congestive heart failure after correction of secondary mitral regurgitation in end-stage cardiomyopathy. Am Heart J 129:1165–1170

7. Batista R (1999) Partial left ventriculectomy – the Batista procedure. Eur J Cardio-Thorac Surg 15(Suppl 1):S12–S19

8. Batista RJ, Santos JL, Takeshita N, Bocchino L, Lima PN, Cunha MA (1996) Partial left ventriculectomy to improve left ventricular function in end-stage heart disease. J Card Surg 11(2):96–97

9. Batista RJV, Verde J, Nery P, Bocchino L, Takeshita N, Bhayana JN, Bergsland J, Graham S, Houck JP, Salerno TA (1997) Partial left ventriculectomy to treat end-stage heart disease. Ann Thorac Surg 64:634–638

10. Blondheim DS, Jacobs LE, Kotler MN, Costacurta GA, Parry WR (1991) Dilated cardiomyopathy with mitral regurgitation: decreased survival despite a low frequency of left ventricular thrombus. Am Heart J 122(3 pt 1):763–771

11. Blum A, Miller H (1998) Role of cytokines in heart failure. Am Heart J 135(2 pt 1):181–186

12. Bohm M (1998) Catecholamine refractoriness and their mechanisms in cardiocirculatory shock and chronic heart failure. J Thorac Cardiovasc Surg 46(Suppl): 270–276

13. Bohm M (1995) Alterations of beta-adrenoceptor-G-protein-regulated adenylyl cyclase in heart failure. Mol Cell Biochem 147(1–2):147–160

14. Bohm M, Diet F, Kemkes B, Erdmann E (1998) Enhancement of the effectiveness of milrinone to increase force of contraction by stimulation of cardiac beta-adrenoceptors in the failing human heart. Klinische Wochenschrift 66(19):957–962

15. Bolling SF, Deeb GM, Brunsting LA, Bach DS (1995) Early outcome of mitral valve reconstruction in patients with end-stage cardiomyopathy. J Thorac Cardiovasc Surg 109(4):676–683

16. Bolling SF, Pagani FD, Deeb GM, Bach SF (1998) Intermediate-term outcome of mitral reconstruction in cardiomyopathy. J Thorac Cardiovasc Surg 115:381–388

17. Boltwood CM, Tei C, Wong M, Shah PM (1983) Quantitative echocardiography of the mitral complex in dilated cardiomyopathy: the mechanism of functional mitral regurgitation. Circulation 68(3):498–508

18. Bristow MR, Ginsburg R, Minobe W, Cubicciotti RS, Sageman WS, Lurie K, Billingham ME, Harrison DE, Stinson EB (1982) Decreased catecholamine sensitivity and beta-adrenergic receptor density in failing human hearts. N Engl J Med 307:205–211

19. Brodde OE (1991) Beta 1- and Beta 2-adrenoceptors in the human heart: properties, function, and alterations in chronic heart failure. Pharmacol Rev 43(2):203–242

20. Chandraratna PA, Aronow WS (1981) Mitral valve ring in normal vs. dilated left ventricle. Cross-sectional echocardiographic study. Chest 79(2):151–154

21. Chen FY, Adams DH, Aranki SF, Collins JJ, Couper GS, Rizzo RJ, Cohn LH (1998) Mitral valve repair in cardiomyopathy. Circulation 98:II-124–II-127

22. David TE, Uden DE, Strauss HD (1983) The importance of the mitral apparatus in left ventriuclar function after correction of mitral regurgitation. Circulation 68(3 pt 2):II76–1182
23. Dowling RD, Koenig S, Laureano A, Cerrito P, Gray LA (1998) Results of partial left ventriculectomy in patients with end-stage idiopathic dilated cardiomyopathy. J Heart Lung Transplant 17:1208–1212
24. Dreyfus GD, Duboc D, Blasco A, Vigoni F, Dubois C, Brodaty D, deLentdecker P, Bachet J, Goudot B, Guilmet D (1994) Myocardial viability assessment in ischemic cardiomyopathy: benefits of coronary revascularization. Ann Thorac Surg 57:1402–1408
25. Fann JI, Ingels NB, Miller DC (1997) Pathophysiology of mitral valve disease and operative indications. In: Edmunds LH (ed) Cardiac Surgery in the Adult. McGraw-Hill, NY, pp 959–990
26. Feldman MD, Copelas L, Gwathmey JK, Phillips P, Warren SE, Schoen FJ, Grossman W, Morgan JP (1987) Deficient production of cyclic AMP: pharmacologic evidence of an important cause of contractile dysfunction in patients with end-stage heart failure. Circulation 75(2):331–339
27. Ferrari R, Bachetti T, Confortini R, Opasich C, Febo O, Corti A, Cassani G, Visioli O (1995) Tumor necrosis factor soluble receptors in patients with various degrees of congestive heart failure. Circulation 92(6):1479–1486
28. Frazier OH (1994) First use of an untethered, vented electric left ventricular assist device for long-term support. Circulation 89(6):2908–2914
29. Gallino A, Jenni R, Hurni R, Hirzel HO, Krayenbuhl HP, Egloff L, Rothlin M, Schonbeck M, Turina M (1987) Early results after mitral valvuloplasty for pure mitral regurgitation. Eur Heart J 8(8):902–905
30. Goldman ME, Mora F, Guarino T, Fuster V, Mindich BP (1987) Mitral valvuloplasty is superior to valve replacement for preservation of left ventricular function: an intraoperative two-dimensional echocardiographic study. J Am Coll Cardiol 10(3):568–575
31. Goldstein DJ, Oz MC, Rose EA (1998) Medical progress: implantable left ventricular assist devices. NEJM 339(21):1522–1533
32. Gorcsan J, Feldman AM, Kormos RL, Mandarino WA, Demetris AJ, Batista RJ (1998) Heterogeneous immediate effects of partial left ventriculectomy on cardiac performance. Circulation 97(9):839–842
33. Hagewisch S, Weh HJ, Hossfeld DK (1990) TNF-induced cardiomyopathy. Lancet 335(8684):294–295
34. Harding SE, Brown LA, Wynne DG, Davies CH, Poole-Wilson PA (1994) Mechanisms of β-adrenoceptor desensitization in the failing human heart. Cardiovasc Res 28:1451–1460
35. Herrera-Garza EH, Stetson SJ, Cubillos-Garzon A, Vooletich MT, Farmer JA, Torre-Amione G (1999) Tumor necrosis factor-α: A mediator of disease progression in the failing human heart. Chest 115:1170–1174
36. Huikuri HV (1983) Effect of mitral valve replacement on left ventricular function in mitral regurgitation. Br Heart J 49(4):328–333
37. Hunt SA (1998) Current status of cardiac transplantation. JAMA 280(19):1692–1698
38. Izumi S, Miyatake K, Beppu S, Park YD, Nagata S, Kinoshita N, Sakakibara H, Nimura Y (1987) Mechanism of mitral regurgitation in patients with myocardial infarction: a study using real-time two-dimensional Doppler flow imaging and echocardiography. Circulation 76(4):777–785
39. Juilliere Y, Danchin N, Briancon S, Khalife K, Ethevenot G, Balaud A, Gilgenkrantz JM, Pernot C, Cherrier F (1988) Dilated cardiomyopathy: long-term follow-up and predictors of survival. Int J Cardiol 21(3):269–277

40. Kay GL, Kay JH, Zubiate P, Yokoyama T, Mendez M (1986) Mitral valve repair for mitral regurgitation secondary to coronary artery disease. Circulation 74(3 pt 2):188–198

41. Kawaguchi HK, Kitabatake A (1997) Alterations of signal transduction system in heart failure. Japan Heart J 38:317–332

42. Konertz W, Khoynezhad A, Sidiropoulos A, Borak V, Baumann G (1999) Early and intermediate results of left ventricular reduction surgery. Eur J Cardio-thorac Surg 15(Suppl 1): S26–S30

43. Kono T, Sabbah HN, Rosman H, Alam M, Jafri S, Goldstein S (1992) Left ventricular shape is the primary determinant of functional mitral regurgitation in heart failure. J Am Coll Cardiol 20(7):1594–1598

44. Levine B, Kalman J, Mayer L, Fillit HM, Packer M (1990) Elevated circulating levels of tumor necrosis factor in severe chronic heart failure. N Engl J Med 323:236–241

45. Magovern JA, Magovern GJ, Maher TD, Benckart DH, Park SB, Christlieb IY, Magovern GJ (1993) Operation for congestive heart failure: transplantation, coronary artery bypass, and cardiomyoplasty. Ann Thorac Surg 56:418–425

46. McCarthy JF, McCarthy PM, Starling RC, Smedira NG, Scalia GM, Wong J, Kasirajan V, Goormastic M, Young JB (1998) Partial left ventriculectomy and mitral valve repair for end-stage congestive heart failure. Eur J Cardio-thorac Surg 13:337–343

47. Milani RV, Mehra MR, Endres S, Eigler A, Cooper ES, Lavie CJ, Ventura HO (1996) The clinical relevance of circulating tumor necrosis factor-alpha in acute decompensated chronic heart failure without cachexia. Chest 110(4):992–995

48. Moreira LFP, Jatene AD (1991) Cardiomyoplasty in dilated cardiomyopathy. In: Carpentier A, Chachques JC, Grandjean PA (eds) Cardiomyoplasty. Futura, Armonk, NY, pp 171–183

49. Moreira LFP, Stolf NAG, Bocchi EA, Bacal F, Giorgi MC, Parga JR, Jatene AD (1998) Partial left ventriculectomy with mitral valve preservation in the treatment of patients with dilated cardiomyopathy. J Thorac Cardiovasc Surg 115:800–807

50. Nagatsu M, Ishihara K, Zile MR, Tsutsui H, Tagawa H, DeFreyte G, Tanaka R, Cooper G, Carabello BA (1994) The effects of complete versus incomplete mitral valve repair in experimental mitral regurgitation. J Thorac Cardiovasc Surg 107(2):416–423

51. Pagani FD, Baker LS, Hsi C, Knox M, Fink MP, Visner MS (1992) Left ventricular systolic and diastolic dysfunction after infusion of tumor necrosis factor-a in conscious dogs. J Clin Invest 90:389–398

52. Pennington DG, Swartz MT, Lohmann DP, McBride LR (1998) Cardiac assist devices. Surgical Clinics of North America 78(5):691–704

53. Phillips HR, Levine FH, Carter JE, Boucher CA, Osbakken MD, Okada RD, Akins CW, Daggett WM, Buckley MJ, Pohost GM (1981) Mitral valve replacement for isolated mitral regurgitation: analysis of clinical course and late postoperative left ventricular ejection fraction. Am J Cardiol 48(4):647–654

54. Pinson CW, Cobanoglu A, Metwdorff MT, Grunkemeier GL, Kay PH, Starr A (1984) Late surgical results for ischemic mitral regurgitation. Role of wall motion score and severity of regurgitation. J Thorac Cardiovasc Surg 88(5 pt 1):663–672

55. Pitarys CJ II, Forman MB, Panayiotou H, Hansen DE (1990) Long-term effects of excision of the mitral apparatus on global and regional ventricular function in humans. J Am Coll Cardiol 15(3):557–563

56. Rankin JS, Feneley MP, Hickey MS, Muhlbaier LH, Wchsler AS, Floyd RD, Reves JG, Skelton TN, Califf RM, Lowe JE (1988) A clinical comparison of mitral valve repair versus replacement in ischemic mitral regurgitation. J Thorac Cadiovasc Surg 95(2):165–177

57. Rosario LB, Stevenson LW, Solomon SD, Lee RT, Reimold SC (1998) The mechanism of decrease in dynamic mitral regurgitation during heart failure treatment: importance of reduction in the regurgitant orifice size. J Am Coll Cardiol 32:1819–1824
58. Salerno TA, Bhayana J (1997) Volume reduction surgery in the treatment of end-stage heart diseases. In: Karp RB, Laks H, Wechsler AS (eds) Advances in Cardiac Surgery, Vol 9. Mosby-Year Book, St. Louis, pp 87–97
59. Sarris GE, Cahill PD, Hansen DE, Derby GC, Miller DC (1988) Restoration of left ventricular systolic performance after reattachment of the mitral chordae tendineae. The importance of valvular-ventricular interaction. J Thorac Cadiovasc Surg 95(6):969–979
60. Schuler G, Peterson KL, Johnson A, Francis G, Dennish G, Utley J, Daily PO, Ashburn W, Ross J Jr (1979) Temporal response of left ventricular performance to mitral valve surgery. Circulation 59(6):1218–1231
61. Stevenson LW, Fowler MB, Schroeder JS, Stevenson WG, Dracup KA, Fond V (1987) Poor survival of patients with idiopathic cardiomyopathy considered too well for transplantation. Am J of Medicine 83(5):871–876
62. Suffredini AF, Fromm RE, Parker MM, Brenner M, Kovacs JA, Wesley RA, Parrillo JE (1989) The cardiovascular response of normal humans to the administration of endotoxin. N Engl J Med 321(26):1828–1830
63. Tavazzi L (1997) Epidemiology of dilated cardiomyopathy: a still undetermined entity. Eur Heart J 18(1):4–6
64. Tischler MD, Cooper KA, Rowen M, LeWinter MM (1994) Myocardial function/valvular heart disease/hypertensive heart disease: mitral valve replacement versus mitral valve repair: a Doppler and quantitative stress echocardiographic study. Circulation 89(1):132–137
65. Torre-Amione G (1999) The syndrome of heart failure: emerging concepts in the understanding of its pathogenesis and treatment. Current Opinion in Cardiology 14:193–195
66. Torre-Amione G, Kapadia S, Benedict C, Oral H, Young JB, Mann DL (1996) Proinflammatory cytokine levels in patients with depressed left ventricular ejection fraction: a report from the Studies of Left Ventricular Dysfunction (SOLVD). J Am Coll Cardiol 27(5):1201–1206
67. Torre-Amione G, Kapadia S, Lee, J, Durand JB, Bies R, Young JB, Mann DL (1996) Tumor necrosis factor-alpha and tumor necrosis factor receptors in the failing human heart. Circulation 93(4):704–711
68. Van Zee KJ, Kohno T, Fischer E, Rock CS, Moldawer LL, Lowry SF (1992) Tumor necrosis factor soluble receptors circulate during experimental and clinical inflammation and can protect against excessive tumor necrosis factor alpha in vitro and in vivo. Proc Nat Acad Sci 89(11):4845–4849
69. Yoran C, Yellin EL, Becker RM, Gabbay S, Frater RW, Sonnenblick EH (1979) Dynamic aspects of acute mitral regurgitation: effects of ventricular volume, pressure and contractility on the effective regurgitant orifice area. Circulation 60(1):170–176

Author's address:

Steven F. Bolling, MD
The University of Michigan
Section of Cardiac Surgery
Taubman Health Care Center, 2120D, Box 0348
1500 E Medical Center Drive
Ann Arbor, Michigan, 48109-0348, USA
E-mail: sbolling@umich.edn

CHAPTER 9 Reduction ventriculoplasty

R. J. V. BATISTA

The principle of reduction ventriculoplasty is based on Nature's law shaping the heart for 100 million years. The snake heart is very tiny, and if it is placed beside a human heart and a buffalo heart, you will see that on a transverse cut they looked exactly the same except for their sizes (Fig. 1). If a computer image of the snake heart is enlarged to the size of the buffalo heart you can no longer say which is which (Fig. 2). The ratio of mass to diameter is the same for all hearts. I even dared to formulate this as $M = 4 \cdot R^3$ (M heart muscle mass; R heart radius). In this example, the coral snake heart has a 1 cm diameter and 5 gr of muscle. A human heart is 10 times larger but has 100 times more muscle mass and the buffalo heart is 10 times greater in diameter but has 1000 times more mass than the tiny coral snake heart. Linear growth in size is accompanied with exponential growth in muscle mass (Fig. 3). Reversing that means that a small reduction in size will compensate for a great amount of muscle mass. In other words, it is much easier to restore the "normal" relationship diameter/ mass by reducing the diameter than by adding functioning mass to a given heart. And this is exactly how reduction ventriculoplasty (RVP) works.

In normal hearts, the left ventricular cavity exists only in the beating heart. We can see and measure it by echocardio- and angiography. Once

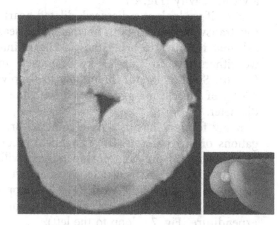

Fig. 1. Buffalo heart (left) and snake's heart (right)

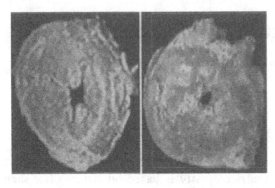

Fig. 2. Muscle mass to cavum ratio in buffalo (left) and snake heart (right)

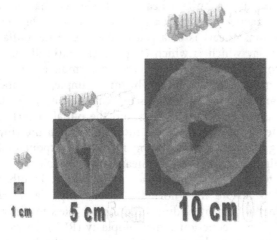

Fig. 3. Heart radius and muscle mass proportions in (left to right) snake, human, buffalo

you dissect a non-living animal heart you see that the ventricle has almost a virtual cavity (Fig. 4).

Now if we look at a diseased, dilated heart (Fig. 5) and make a comparative transverse cut for both normal and diseased heart, we can easily establish that in order to bring the sick heart into shape with the normal one, we either have to add 3.5 kg of muscle to it or decrease its diameter (Fig. 6). Since it is still impossible to supply the heart with an additional 3.5 kg of muscle mass we are left with the "easier" option: decreasing its diameter.

Many foreign scientists have come to Brasil to make additional investigations on my patients. Dr. Kawaguchi recorded pressure-volume loops in 32 patients [13] pre- and postoperatively with special catheters, introduced directly into the left ventricle. Preoperatively the heart was using a lot of energy to produce little work (Fig. 7 – loop to the right). After a surgical reduction in size, the "new" heart did more work with much less energy expenditure (Fig. 7 – loop to the left).

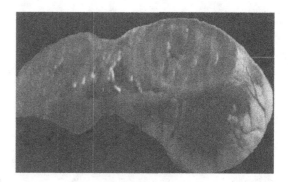

Fig. 4. Almost no cavity is seen in buffalo heart

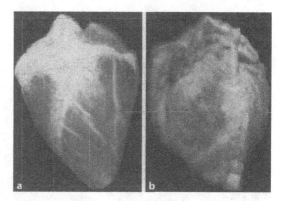

Fig. 5. Normal (**a**) and dilated (**b**) human heart

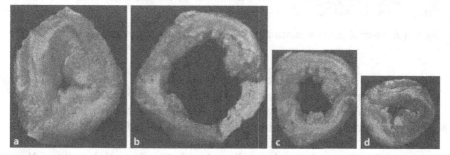

Fig. 6. Transverse cuts through **a** normal heart with the same diameter as **b** dilated heart; **c** and **d** hearts with diameter reduced

Prof. Lunkenheimer [16] measured the wall tension in 17 patients by inserting needle force probes into up to five sites of the left ventricular wall before and after RVP. Focal mesh tension dropped significantly by 40 ± 22% after RVP (Fig. 8).

Many surgeons also came to see the procedure performed and observe the patients postoperatively. Alternatively, I visited many of them in their

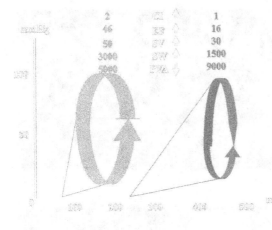

Fig. 7. Pressure/volume curves – pre-operatively (right curve) and after PVR (left curve)

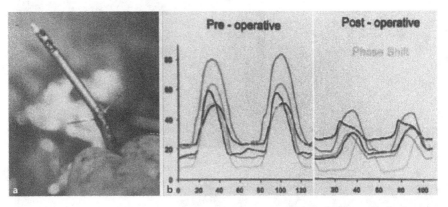

Fig. 8. a Wall tension probes in myocardium; **b** wall tension curves pre- and postoperatively

countries to perform the procedure in their hospitals – this way teaching them and spreading the knowledge. All this eventually led to an increased number of RVP performed worldwide. The results have been presented many times on different occasions and at specially dedicated forums [2–5]. Some of these could be summarized as follows:

The Buffalo General Hospital affiliated with The State University of New York was the first to recognize our work, and Prof. Salerno [7] started the first program of partial left ventriculectomy in North America in June 1995. From all the patients (28 patients through 1997), who were preoperatively in NYHA class III–IV and all but one not accepted for heart transplantation, 60% left the hospital in class I after RVP. At present, Prof. Salerno's experience includes 45 patients with 85% hospital survival.

Profs. P. McCarthy and R. Starling [17] from the Cleveland Clinic also came to Brazil and started to perform RVP thereafter. In 62 patients they have had a 1.2% hospital mortality and 80% of those who survived 1 year

(87% actuarial survival) were in NYHA class I (Fig. 9). These results are similar to the results of effected heart transplantation in one year but much better than the cumulated mortality from the waiting list and transplanted patients (70% actuarial survival rate in one year; Fig. 10). They have treated only patients with cardiomyopathy and no coronary artery disease.

Similar results have been demonstrated by Prof. R. Dowling from the Jewish Hospital in Louisville [10] with 16 patients with RVP versus 17 transplanted.

Meanwhile, we tried to prove whether these results are due to a ventricular diameter reduction or to the mitral valve repair. A series of 20 patients was treated differently: first a mitral valve repair was done, patient

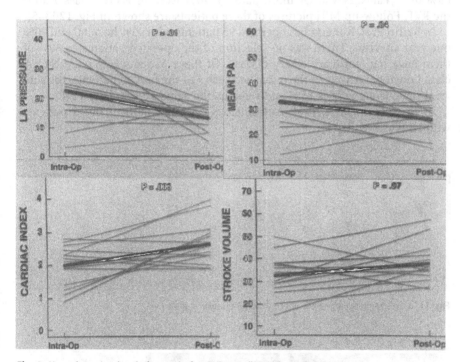

Fig. 9. Hemodynamics data before and after RVP as collected by McCarthy

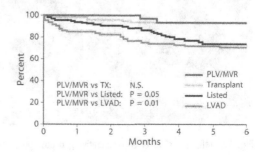

Fig. 10. Actuarial survival after RVP, VAD and heart transplantation based on data from McCarthy

taken off the bypass and cardiac function evaluated. All the patients in this series had a worsening of ventricular function and 80% required inotropes to come off bypass. Then we went back on bypass and performed the RVP. Coming off bypass thereafter was much easier and only 20% required inotropes. Their ejection fraction improved. These series showed that the ventricular function improves with diameter reduction only (Fig. 11).

Adding the ventricular function improvement by RVP to the chronic left ventricular unloading by the left ventricular assisting device (LVAD), H. Frazier from the Texas Heart Institute was able to wean two patients from LVAD [11].

In Japan Prof. H. Suma has operated 45 patients with 90% hospital and 85% one year survival. Of those patients 70% were in NYHA class I after the RVP. Follow-up MRI pictures of these patients are shown in Fig. 12 [3–5].

In Berlin Prof. Konertz has operated 95 patients with 95% hospital and 90% one year survival. There was no selection of the operated patients as 80% of them have had coronary artery disease. Of these patients 80% were NYHA class I postoperatively. In the published series of the first 30 patients, the survival rate at one year is 85% and remains the same 3 years later [14].

In Bristol, England, Prof. Angelini has operated more than 30 patients with similar results [1].

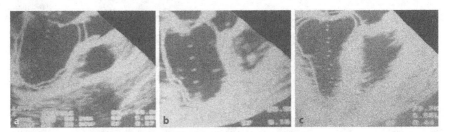

Fig. 11. a LV size preoperatively; **b** after mitral valve repair; **c** after RVP

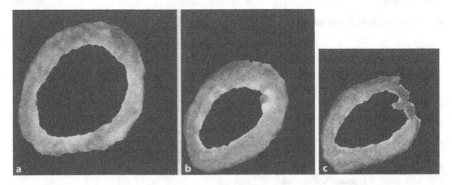

Fig. 12. MRI "slices" of LV **a** preoperatively; **b** postoperatively and **c** one year later

In Belgrad (Prof. Gradinac) and in Taiwan (Prof. T. Yen) and Indonesia (Prof. H. Tarmisi) 22, 15, and 11 patients, respectively, have been operated and their results are very similar – 85% hospital and 68% one year survival and 80% in NYHA class I [5, 12].

In Brazil there are already several centers performing PVR. Prof. F. Luchese from Porto Alegre was the first one to apply the principle of LV diameter reduction and to operate several patients [15]. He was able to obtain a significant reduction of the pulmonary vascular resistance after RVP in two patients.

In Coracao, Bellotti et al. operated and investigated 11 patients. Hospital survival was 100%. The 6-month and 4-year survivals were the same – 60%; and 70% were in NYHA class I postoperatively. They demonstrated that the ventricles become thicker postoperatively which in turn improves EF even more [6]. They correlated mortality with myocite thickness and found out that in patients with a myocite thickness of more than 22 μm mortality is significantly higher [9].

Dr. Bombonato [8], working in a small town in the Amazon, also presented good results with 7 patients at the cardiac surgery meeting in Fortaleza.

Our own results are based on 720 patients operated between 1983 and 1999. Seventy percent were males and their age varied between 6 months and 95 years with a mean of 46 years. These patients were in NYHA class IV preoperatively with an EF of less than 18% measured by echocardiography. Some of them were taken to the operating room under cardiac massage.

Most common pathology leading to cardiac dilation in these patients was coronary disease in 30%; valvular disease – in 20%; postviral cardiomyopathy – in 20%; idiopathic cardiomyopathy – in 20%; Chagas disease – in 5%; and others – in 5%.

Postoperatively their EF improved by 100–300% as estimated by transesophageal echo and in some by DSA. Their clinical condition improved significantly – 60% became NYHA class I; 30% – class II; and 10% – class III. Most common postoperative complications were renal failure – 20%; arrhythmias – 15%; bleeding – 10%; and others – 5%. Operating room survival was 95% and hospital survival 85%. One year after the operation the survival rate was 65%; two years – 60%; 3 years – 57%; and 4 years – 55%.

All these patients, which I operated in Brazil, should have been dead within 6 months without this alternative to an expensive and generally not available treatment modality like heart transplantation. Thus, lack of medical facilities to help the very sick Brasilian patients stimulated me to develop a simple, inexpensive method to treat terminally ill patients with reasonably good chances for a better quality of life.

■ References

1. Angelini GD et al (1997) The Batista procedure for end stage heart failure. Lancet 350:489
2. Batista RJ (1995) First symposium "Batista Procedure"; Lima, Peru

3. Batista RJ (1996) Second symposium "The Batista Procedure"; Tokyo, Japan
4. Batista RJ (1997) Third symposium "Batista Procedure"; Chietti, Italy
5. Batista RJ (1998) Fourth symposium "Batista Procedure"; Kyoto, Japan
6. Bellotti G, Moraes A, Bocchi E, Esteves FA, Stolf N, Bacal F, Medeiros C, Graziosi P, Cerri G, Jatene A, Pileggi F (1997) Efeitos da Ventriculectomia Parcial nas propriedades mecanicas, forma e geometria do VE em pacientes con miocardiopathia dilatada. [Effects of partial ventriculectomy on left ventricular mechanical properties, shape, and geometry in patients with dilated cardiomyopathy]. Arq Bras de Cardiol 67:395–400
7. Bergsland J, Batista RJV, Hasnain S, Houck J, Graham S, Bhayana J, Salerno TA (1998) The Buffalo experience – partial left ventriculectomy. In: Kawaguchi AT, Linde LM (eds) Partial Left Ventriculectomy. Its Theory, Results and Perspectives. Excerpta Medica
8. Bombonato R, Bestetti RB, Sgarbieri R, Kato M, Caixe SH, Moreira Neto FF, Finzi LA, Brasil JC (1996) Experiencia inicial com a ventriculectomia parcial esquerda no tratamento da insuficiencia cardiaca terminal. [Initial experience with partial left ventriculectomy as a treatment for end-stage heart failure]. Arch Bras Cardiologia 66:189–192
9. Congresso Brasileiro de Cirurgia Cardiaca, Porto Alegre, 1994
10. Etoch SW, Koenig SC, Laureano MA, Cerrito P, Gray LA, Dowling RD (1999) Results after partial left ventriculectomy versus heart transplantation for idiopathic cardiomyopathy. J Thorac Cardiovasc Surg 117:952–959
11. Frazier OH, Benedict CR, Radovancevic B, Bick RJ, Capek P, Springer WE, Macris MP, Delgado R, Buja LM (1996) Improved left ventricular function after chronic left ventricular unloading. Ann Thorac Surg 62:675–681
12. Gradinac S, Miric M, Popovic AD, Neskovic AN, Jovovic L, Vuk L, Bojic M (1998) Ann Thorac Surg 66:1963–1968
13. Kawaguchi AT, Sugimachi M, Sunagawa K, Ujiie T, Shimura S, Takeshita N, Koide S, Batista RJV (1998) Pre- and postoperative left ventricular pressure-volume relationships in patients undergoing partial left ventriculectomy. In: Kawaguchi AT, Linde LM (eds) Partial Left Ventriculectomy. Its Theory, Results and Perspectives. Excerpta Medica
14. Konertz W, Khoynezhad A, Sidoropoulos A, Borak V, Baumann G (1999) Early and intermediate results of left ventricular reduction surgery. Eur J Cardiothorac Surg 15 (Suppl 1):S 26–30
15. Luchese F et al (1997) Ventriculectomia parcial esquerda: ponte para trasplantante em pacientes insuficiencia cardiaca refrataria e hipertensao pulmonar. Rev Bras de Cir Cardiovasc 12:221
16. Lunkenheimer PP, Redmann K, Cryer CW, Batista RJV, Nery de Lima PR, Salerno TA (1998) Wall stress measured before and after ventriculectomy. In: Kawaguchi AT, Linde LM (eds) Partial Left Ventriculectomy. Its Theory, Results and Perspectives. Excerpta Medica
17. McCarthy PM, Starling RC, Wong J, Scalia GM, Buda T, Vargo RL, Goormastic M, Thomas JD, Smedira NS, Young JB (1997) Early results with partial left ventriculectomy. J Thorac Cardiovasc Surg 114:755

Author's address:

Randas J. Vilela Batista, MD
Vilela Batista Heart Foundation
Rua Carlos Razera # 8
Curitiba – Brazil – 80.810.310

CHAPTER 10

Artificial heart:
today's facts and future horizons

A. El-Banayosy and R. Körfer

■ Milestones

One year before Barnard inaugurated the era of cardiac transplantation, DeBakey for the first time successfully applied a left ventricular bypass pump for temporary circulatory assistance in a patient with postcardiotomy heart failure [1]. In 1969, Cooley was the first to apply a total artificial heart [2]. However, it took almost ten more years before a successful bridge-to-transplant procedure could be reported [3]. In 1982, DeVries for the first time implanted a Jarvik 100 total artificial heart for permanent use, which soon turned out to be unsuccessful and represented a major set-back for the dream of an artificial heart [4].

The early 1980's brought the breakthrough of cyclosporine significantly improving the outcome after heart transplantation. As a consequence, the demand in heart-assist devices, particularly as a bridge to transplantation, was renewed with several devices being put on the market during the following years. One of these was the Novacor LVAS, which in 1984 was successfully employed in a patient prior to cardiac transplantation [5]. In 1988, the Frazier group was the first to implant the HeartMate left ventricular assist device (Thermo Cardiosystems) [6]. Another major milestone was the development of the wearable Novacor LVAS, which allowed the patient to be fully ambulant and even to be discharged home with the device [7, 8]. Some patients were even able to return to work while being supported with the Novacor LVAS. Another milestone was the first clinical implantation of the miniaturized DeBakey axial flow pump in 1999.

In the meantime, several devices have become available, which allow the patient to be discharged home while on support under certain circumstances, thus enjoying an almost normal life while waiting for cardiac transplantation. The application of mechanical circulatory support as an alternative to transplantation is within reach.

■ Heart Center experience

Since 1987, 438 patients (345 men, 93 women, mean age 52 years) have received mechanical circulatory support at our institution with 474 implantations being performed. Table 1 details the number of patients as to indication, with "miscellaneous" including cardiogenic shock for various reasons

Table 1. Indications for mechanical circulatory support

	Extracorporeal systems (n = 199)*	Paracorporeal systems (n = 143)	Implantable systems (n = 127)
Postcardiotomy heart failure	124	21	2
BTT	29	104	113
Miscellaneous	46	18	12

* 5 patients of this group received both the Biomedicus and the Abiomed device

such as myocarditis, acute myocardial infarction, right heart failure, acute rejection primary graft failure, alternative to transplantation, and bridge to recovery.

At present, six different systems are in clinical use at our center. The extracorporeal devices, the Biomedicus centrifugal pump (n = 122), and the Abiomed BVS 5000 (n = 82) are used for short-term support mainly in patients with postcardiotomy heart failure, with right heart failure following cardiac transplantation, or in combination with an implantable left ventricular assist device. During our initial experience, the centrifugal pump was also applied for bridging patients to transplantation; some of them had postcardiotomy heart failure which turned out to be irreversible. The device was used for left ventricular assistance in 106 patients, for right ventricular assistance in 12 patients, and for biventricular support in 81 patients. Five patients had to be supported with both devices. In 49 cases, the device was used as a femoral-femoral cardiopulmonary bypass. Duration of support in this collective was 1 hour to 28 days (5 ± 4 days).

The devices located in paracorporeal position are the Thoratec VAD (n = 135) and the Medos HIA-VAD (n = 8), preferably employed for medium-term support. The Thoratec system is mainly applied for biventricular assistance in patients bridged to cardiac transplantation. Both devices are used for right ventricular support in addition to left ventricular support by an implantable system. Moreover, the Medos HIA-VAD can also be applied in children, because it is available in different sizes. 69 patients each received biventricular and left ventricular support, 5 patient right ventricular assistance. Duration of support was 2–367 days (47 ± 52 days).

The most recent generation of mechanical circulatory support systems available at our institution are the implantable devices Novacor LVAS (n = 79) and VE HeartMate (n = 48); both are for long-term left ventricular assistance in patients bridged to cardiac transplantation and are an alternative to transplantation. Duration of support was 8 hours to 800 days (134 ± 147 days). Figures 1 and 2 provide a survey on the systems applied with regard to indication and kind of support.

Main complications occurring under support were bleeding, infection, and thromboembolism. The outcomes of all patients are described in detail in Table 2.

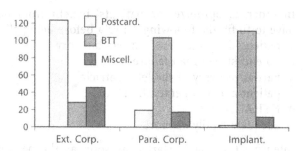

Fig. 1. Systems applied with regard to indication

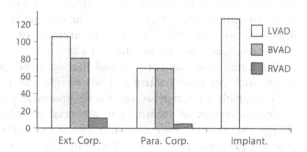

Fig. 2. Systems applied with regard to kind of support

Table 2. Results of 469 implantations of mechanical circulatory support systems at the Heart Center NRW

Outcome	Extracorporeal systems (n = 199)	Paracorporeal systems (n = 143)	Implantable systems (n = 127)
Weaned	80	5	4
Transplanted	29	72	59
Waiting	1	8	15
Discharged	68 (34.3%)	67 (49.6%)	54 (48.2%)

▦ Out-of-hospital (OOH) experience

One of the decisive advantages of the implantable devices is the option of discharging patients under support. Our initial objectives were to allow patients to live a near-normal life on LVAD support, to free-up hospital resources, to reduce costs of long ICU stays, and to advance the alternative-to-transplant potential of LVAD therapy. On the basis of five years of MCS experience, we established protocols for the selection of patients participating in our OOH program, for their home management, and for their long-term follow-up. A VAD team consisting of a cardiac surgeon, a cardiologist, an intensivist, and two VAD coordinators is responsible for patient selection and management.

In order to optimize the patients' benefit from our OOH program, they have to fulfill the following criteria before being allowed to go home:
■ patients fully recovered and ambulatory
■ no end-stage organ failure
■ partial recovery of the left ventricle
■ patient able to operate the LVAD
■ NYHA I status
■ adequate family support

Intensive training is started as soon as the patients are moved from the ICU to the ward. Patient and family members are taught how to operate the LVAD system under routine conditions as well as how to troubleshoot when conditions are irregular. Additionally, patients learn to perform various tests such as INR self-test, measurement of blood pressure and body temperature, and to care for the exit site.

The home management protocol that we developed for this patient collective includes daily control of body weight and INR (self-test), and twice daily controls of temperature, blood pressure, pump output, as well as wound redressement according to a special protocol. Four weeks after discharge the patient returns to our center for follow-up which includes a physical examination, echocardiography, chest X-ray (not mandatory), exit site inspection and redressement, laboratory diagnosis, Swan-Ganz catheterization, and stress tests (optional). Moreover, the patient and his family members have the opportunity to discuss any problems associated with the device with the VAD team. Then, 8–12 weeks later, the patient again presents himself for PET scanning and Swan-Ganz catheterization, echocardiography, and stress testing to evaluate the recovery of the heart.

Sixty-two LVAD patients (54 men, 8 women, age 51 ± 12 years, 44 Novacor, 18 HeartMate) fulfilled our criteria for being discharged home while on support. They were supported for 1–755 days (mean 153 ± 167 days); 43 Novacor patients and 28 HeartMate patients had to be readmitted to the hospital for mainly neurological disorders and infections. However, our OOH experience with these patients was encouraging and proved the safety and reliability of this technology. Some of these patients even returned to work while on support. They have worked as a saleswoman in a butchery, baker, physician, programmer, farmer, waiter. They are also allowed to start light sports activities except for swimming, and most of them have driven their own car. Hence, quality of life in most of our OOH patients can be described as near normal. The first step toward future horizons has thus been accomplished.

■ Future horizons

In spite of the outstanding progress in the field of mechanical circulatory support, there are still some limitations to wider acceptance and application of this technology. The devices are still bulky, not fully implantable (driveline), not versatile with regard to sizes and kind of support, and are

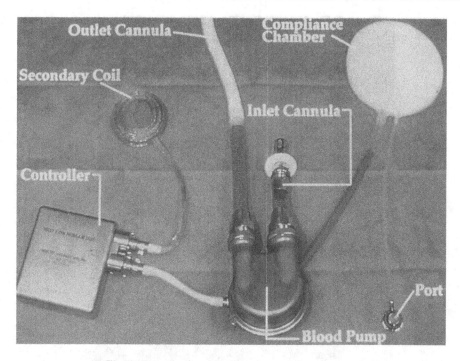

Fig. 3. The LionHeart™ LVD 2000 LVAD

associated with a high morbidity (bleeding, infection, thrombembolism). These shortcomings have resulted in the demands the new generation of systems have to fulfill.

The LionHeart™ LVD 2000 LVAD (Fig. 3) has already been investigated in animal experiments with encouraging results at Penn State University and will be available for the first human implantation by the end of 1999. It consists of external and internal components for operation without percutaneous lines or conduits. The blood pump assembly is electrically powered and is implanted in the preperitoneal space, beneath the left costal margin. It features a motor, a pusher plate mechanism, a smooth blood sac, and two tilting disk valves for unidirectional flow. Connection to the native circulation is achieved via inlet and outlet cannulae.

The motor controller and internal coil control the operation of the blood pump assembly. Controller and blood pump are powered either by external sources or rechargeable batteries located in the controller. External power is received transcutaneously by the internal coil and sent to the motor controller and blood pump assembly for continuous operation. Internal power is delivered by the motor controller's rechargeable batteries and allows the LionHeart™ LVD 2000 LVAD recipient to function totally free of the external power source for approximately 30 minutes. The motor controller is placed under the anterior abdominal wall or in the preperitoneal

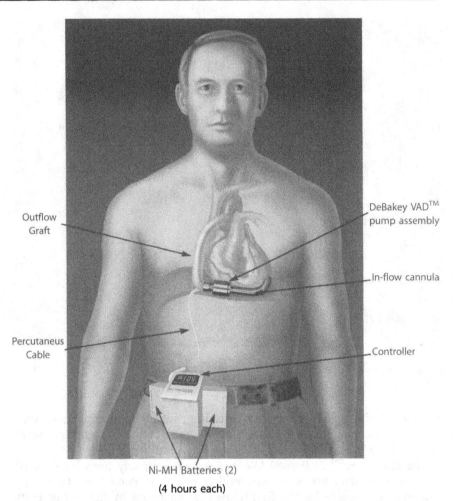

Outflow Graft

DeBakey VAD™ pump assembly

In-flow cannula

Percutaneus Cable

Controller

Ni-MH Batteries (2)
(4 hours each)

Fig. 4. DeBakey VAD™ blood pump (with kind permission of Micromed Technology Inc.)

space, beneath the right costal margin. The internal coil is located in the subcutaneous tissue of the chest wall.

The compliance chamber assembly and access port serve as a gas-volume accumulator. The compliance chamber assembly provides gas to evacuated chambers of the blood pump assembly during its operation. This complicance chamber assembly is placed in the left pleural space, and the access port is passed through the intercostal space and is anchored in the subcutaneous tissue over the left anterior chest wall.

The power transmitter with a coil transfers power across the intact skin. It is connected to the power pack in normal operation, and will likely be worn on a belt or in a pack.

The *DeBakey VAD™* (Fig. 4) is a miniaturized axial flow blood pump, however with external power source. First clinical experiences have been

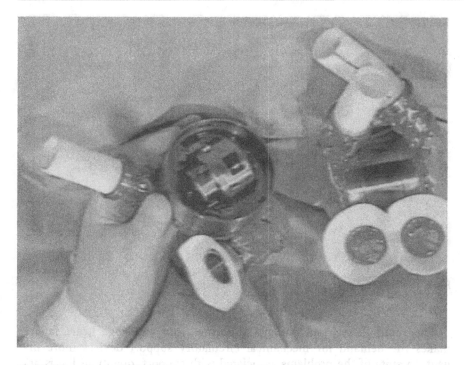

Fig. 5. Abiomed total artificial heart

made in Berlin, Paris, and Vienna, but there were still some minor technical problems.

It consists of three subsystems: a pump system, a controller system, and a clinical data acquisition system (CDAS). The blood pump is an implantable, titanium, electromagnetically actuated axial flow pump. It is 30.5 mm in diameter, 76.2 mm in length, and weighs 93 g. A titanium inflow cannula connects the pump to the ventricular apex and a vascular graft (outflow conduit) connects the pump to the aorta. Blood flow from the pump is measured by a flow probe placed around the outflow conduit. The flow probe's wiring is bundled with the pump motor's wiring in a cable assemly which exits the skin superior to the iliac crest on the right frontal portion of the body and attaches to the VAD's external controller system. The controller system may be connected to the batteries or the external CDAS. The CDAS receives pump speed, flow, power, and current signals from the controller and displays that information so the user can monitor and adjust pump operation.

Another device is the *Abiomed total artificial heart* (Fig. 5), the first electrically driven, fully implantable system of this kind, which is expected to be available by the end of 2000. Another very small device will be the *HeartSaver Canadian Heart* (Fig. 6), which is fully implantable, but only for left ventricular support. Finally, new versions of the Novacor and HeartMate devices are currently being developed.

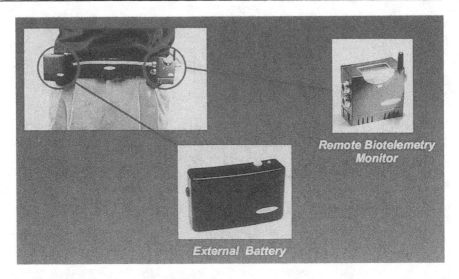

Fig. 6. HeartSaver Canadian Heart

The rapid increase in patients suffering from end-stage heart failure makes the demand for mechanical circulatory support devices more urgent. In spite of the problems associated with support, quality of life is acceptable. Since the new generation of devices has shown promising results in pre-clinical studies, we believe that morbidity associated with this technology can be further reduced. These devices may represent an alternative to transplantation, because in the future, heart transplantation will be restricted to a minority of heart failure patients.

⬛ **Acknowledgments.** We thank the German Association of Organ Recipient (Reg. Ass.) for grant support

⬛ References

1. DeBakey ME (1971) Left ventricular bypass pump for cardiac assistance: clinical experience. Am J Cardiol 27:3–11
2. Cooley DA, Liotta D, Hallman GL et al. (1969) Orthotopic cardiac prosthesis for two-staged cardiac replacement. Am J Cardiol 24:723–730
3. Reemtsma K, Krusin R, Edie R et al. (1978) Cardiac transplantation in patients requiring mechanical circulatory support. N Engl J Med 298:670
4. DeVries WC, Anderson JL, Joyce LD et al. (1984) Clinical use of the total artificial heart. N Engl J Med 310:273–278
5. Starnes VA, Oyer PE, Portner PE (1988) Isolated left ventricular assist as bridge to cardiac transplantation. J Thorac Cardiovasc Surg 96:62–71
6. McGee MG, Myers TJ, Abou-Awdi N et al. (1991) Extended support with a left ventricular assist device as a bridge to heart transplantation. ASAIO Trans 37:M425–426

7. Loisance DY, Leleuze PH, Mazzucotelli JP et al. (1994) Clinical implantation of the wearable Baxter Novacor ventricular assist system. Ann Thorac Surg 58:551–554
8. Kormos RL, Murali S, Dew MA et al. (1994) Chronic mechanical circulatory support: rehabilitation, low morbidity, and superior survival. Ann Thorac Surg 57:51–57

Author's address:

Dr. A. El-Banayosy
Herzzentrum NRW
Klinik für Thorax-
und Kardiovaskularchirurgie
Georgstr. 11
D-32545 Bad Oeynhausen, Germany
E-mail: abanayosy@hdz-nrw.ruhr-uni-bochum.de

CHAPTER 11 Apoptosis in heart failure – reversible?

D. Darmer, B. Bartling, and J. Holtz

The contribution of cardiomyocyte apoptosis to cardiac pathologies such as myocardial infarction and terminal heart failure has been suggested on the basis of histochemical and biochemical demonstrations of apoptotic nuclear DNA fragmentation. However, these techniques have yielded highly different figures of apoptotic myocytes between different laboratories, suggesting that they are not without methodological pitfalls. Apoptotic "melting rates" of myocardial tissue cannot be derived from DNA fragmentation histochemistry. Therefore, the debate on the relevance of myocyte apoptosis is ongoing, although experimental studies with inhibitory interventions into the apoptotic program demonstrate its involvement in ischemia/reperfusion associated myocyte losses and suggest its involvement in overload-induced heart failure. A unique feature of the apoptotic process in failing cardiomyocytes is the "postmitochondrial retardation" of the program: while cytochrome c release from the mitochondria, a critical step in the program, encompasses more than 50% the total myocardial cytochrome c and substantially activates further cytosolic steps of the program, biochemical signs of nucleolysis are still barely detectable and DNA fragmentation histochemistry only stains some 0.2% of the myocytes. It is proposed that this large cytochrome c release impairs mitochondrial respiratory capacity, augments mitochondrial radical formation and activates caspase-mediated degradation of cytosolic proteins involved in signaling and contraction. Therefore, functional impairment due to cytosolic apoptotic processes should be more important for the failing heart than the final irreversible myocyte losses due to nucleolysis. Apoptotic cytochrome c release is a reversible process, provided that the apoptogenic stimulus is removed prior to irreversible nucleolysis. Anecdotal reports in patients with terminal heart failure, in which hemodynamic unloading of the heart by the installation of a ventricular assist device as a bridge to availability of a donor heart was used, demonstrated renormalization of phenotypic features of failing myocardium. In those hearts, several endogenous inhibitors of apoptotic cytochrome c release are upregulated, suggesting that this support partially can reverse the quantitatively important aspect of myocyte apoptosis, the cytosolic activation by cytochrome c release.

▪ Introduction

When the first reports on histologic signs of apoptosis or programmed cell death of cardiomyocytes in several cardiovascular pathologies reached the cardiologic community [for reviews see 11, 16, 32, 35, 56, 67], great expectancies as well as sharp controversies were triggered by these observations. This vivid interest in cardiomyocyte apoptosis and the profound disagreements on its pathophysiological relevance still persist even today [79].

Apoptosis is a genetically determined, highly ritualistic program of active cellular self destruction or suicide, which induces involution of surplus cells and phagocytosis of their remnants by neighboring cells without activation of local or systemic inflammation. The program has been characterized mainly in models of embryologic organ development, in cells of the immune system, and in tumor cells. Several experimental interventions into the program have been developed and have demonstrated that the execution of the suicidal program can be prevented. In view of this background, the expectations which were triggered by reports on a cardiomyocyte apoptosis in severe cardiac diseases appear understandable!

The postulate that myocyte losses by an active apoptotic suicide program contribute to infarct size [3, 37] opens the prospect for salvage of jeopardized myocardium in ischemic heart disease by antiapoptotic preventive treatment. The speculation that distension-induced cardiomyocyte apoptosis [14] is the mechanism mediating the transition from cardiac overload hypertrophy to decompensation and terminal failure [8] yields a highly attractive concept for a still poorly understood process, and a better understanding is the basis for developing better treatment! However, serious doubts about the relevance of cardiomyocyte apoptosis persist, and Table 1 summarizes some of the questions and objections.

Here, we will briefly explain the limitations of the presently available techniques for documentation of myocyte apoptosis in the heart and the still somewhat preliminary arguments for the relevance of the process. Furthermore, we will propose that early, pre-terminal, and still reversible steps of the apoptotic program may have a quantitatively much more important role in overload-associated heart failure than the final apoptotic myocyte losses. We feel that a shift in the discussion from the focus on methodological issues of histologic documentation of nuclear DNA alterations towards a better understanding of the early, reversible steps of the program is more promising.

▪ Histochemical documentation of myocyte death in cardiac tissue

The backbone of the apoptotic program in most cell types is the proteolytic activation of a cascade of cysteine proteases that cleave after aspartic acid residues and which are called caspases [12, 88]. Two major pathways for the activation of the cascade of caspases have been identified: the cell surface death receptor pathway and the pathway initiated by the mitochon-

Table 1. Approaches and problems in identifying apoptotic myocyte death in the heart and in assessing its relevance

Approach	Problem
1) Histochemical documentation of myocyte apoptosis depends on the enzymatic characterization of the type of DNA strand breaks in tissue sections. This is obtained by the TUNEL method [28] or by the Taq polymerase labeling technique [20].	The number of strand breaks required for a positive histochemical "apoptotic" signal is unknown. Such strand breaks also occur in living cells during DNA repair processes [40].
2) Biochemical documentation of apoptotic DNA cleavage requires gel electrophoresis of extracted DNA for showing preferential nucleosome-sized DNA fragmentation [15], see Fig. 2.	Tissue DNA extracts cannot identify the type of cells undergoing nucleosome-sized fragmentation; isolation of a cell type from a tissue after enzymatic cellular dissociation may introduce artefacts; some nucleosome-sized cleavage may also occur in "secondary" necrosis.
3) Apoptotic myocyte nuclei can be identified by electron microscopy (nuclear condensation without major signs of sarcolemmal or mitochondrial damage [58]).	Diagnosis is difficult and may be disturbed by fixation artefacts during preparation of sections [79]. It is extremely labor-intensive to obtain a representative figure of cardiomyocytes identified as apoptotic by electronmicroscopy.
4) Differences in the number of "apoptotic" cardiomyocyte nuclei and/or in an index of nucleosome-sized DNA fragmentation (DNA-"ladder" score [5] are used to demonstrate differences in the apoptotic rate between samples from different hearts.	Reproducible figures of apoptotic cardiomyocyte nuclei cannot yield an estimate of "the rate of myocyte losses" by apoptosis in the tissue, since the "duration" of the histochemical "visibility" of apoptotic DNA cleavage is unknown and cannot be defined. Therefore, histochemistry cannot answer whether myocyte apoptosis is a quantitatively neglectible epiphenomenon or a causal factor in heart pathology.
5) Labor-intensive morphometric assessments of reductions in myocyte number of ventricles in an experimental series may be used to estimate rates of myocyte losses in a certain cardiac pathology.	Cardiomyocyte mitoses do occur in adult mammalian myocardium, and their frequency is enhanced in terminal human heart failure [38]. However, a rate of cardiac myocyte proliferation cannot be obtained from these data, excluding the calculation of a rate of cell losses from comparing morphometrically obtained myocyte numbers.

dria (Fig. 1). In many cell types, apoptosis induced by the death receptor pathway requires the secondary activation of the mitochondrial pathway [44, 78]. The terminal apoptotic steps of the program, induced by the activated effector caspases, include degradation of cytosolic structures and proteins, chromatin condensation, DNA fragmentation, nuclear membrane breakdown, and translocation of phosphatidylserins to the external leaflet of the cell membrane. These latter alterations of the functionally intact cell membranes, which surround shrunken cellular remnants and cytosolic apoptotic bodies, facilitate the non-inflammatory phagocytosis of the remnants by the neighboring cells.

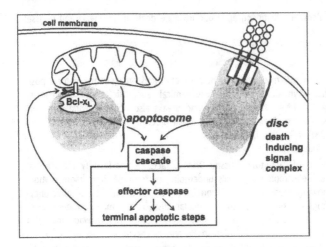

Fig. 1. Two major intracellular signal pathways result in the execution of the terminal steps of the apoptotic program by the cascade of activated caspases:
- Activation of initiator caspases in the signal complex (disc) assembled by many apoptosis-modulating peptides at the death domains of activated death receptors (e.g.: Fas, tumor necrosis factor type I and others).
- Activation of initiator caspases in the apoptosome assembled by apoptosis modulating proteins at the outer mitochondrial membrane; this activation requires release of cytochrome c and ATP from the mitochondria. Release of cytochrome c and activation of caspases is attenuated by antiapoptotic proteins of the Bcl-2 family, such as Bcl-x$_L$, but this inhibition is offset by caspase-mediated cleavage of Bcl-x$_L$

There is general agreement that more than one feature of the program should be identified in dying cells for defining the type of death as apoptotic [15]. However, nuclear DNA alterations (Fig. 2) have been considered as traditional "hallmarks" of apoptosis. Since the discussion on the relevance of apoptosis in the heart focussed on the issue of irreversible myocyte losses, the biochemical and histochemical documentation of these DNA changes became the critical issue. The problems in assessing the relevance of cardiomyocyte apoptosis, listed in Table 1, might suggest that it is impossible to obtain reliable information on cardiac apoptosis. This is certainly a incorrect, exaggerated interpretation!

In the hands of competent, experienced laboratories, the histochemical analyses of cardiomyocyte apoptosis, performed in combination with the use of confocal microscopy for assessments of nuclear morphology, certainly yield quantitative figures with convincing reproducibility between different experimental studies and/or postmortem analyses of human tissues [2, 30, 66, 76, 77]. Parallels between the progression of human heart failure before cardiac transplantation and the frequency of myocyte apoptosis in the explanted ventricles [30, 76] yield a plausible suggestion for a causal contribution of the process to the progression of the disease. Unrealistically high numbers of apoptotic myocyte nuclei in terminally failing

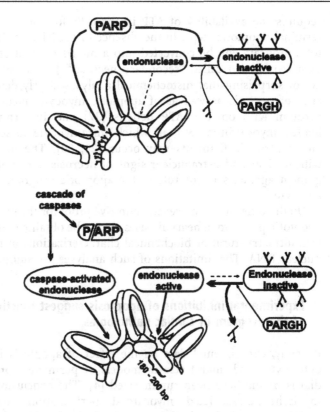

Fig. 2. Apoptotic fragmentation of the DNA into pieces of 180–200 base pairs or multiples thereof results from the arrangement of the DNA helix in "nucleosomes" around histone complexes.
Upper part: This arrangement is stabilized by the poly(ADP-ribose) polymerase (PARP), which protects the nuclear DNA by inactivating nuclear endonucleases and by facilitating repair processes via histone ribosylation. *Lower part:* During apoptosis, caspases inactive PARP by cleavage and liberate a caspase-activated endonuclease for import into the nucleus by cleavage of an inhibitor. In the apoptotic nucleus, the endonucleases attack the DNA mainly between the nucleosomes

human hearts by these histochemcial analyses in the hands of other laboratories [40, 63], partially combined with claims that living myocytes with ongoing DNA repair processes are also labelled as "TUNEL positive" [40], are difficult to explain, as are extremely low numbers reported recently from explanted human hearts [81]. These extreme quantitative differences suggest that the histochemical characterization of apoptotic nuclei in the heart is not without potential pitfalls.

Another much debated problem of biochemical assessment of apoptosis is the critique that nucleosome-sized DNA fragmentation can also occur during necrotic myocyte losses (Table 1, number 2]. This debate may come close to semantic hairsplitting! It is well known from studies in several cell types that the activation of the mitochondrial step in the apoptotic pathway (i.e., release of cytochrome c and other apoptotic signals, see Fig. 1) requires the availability of ATP in the cells for the exact execution of the terminal apoptotic steps. In the absence of sufficient cellular ATP, the apoptotic program will be converted into a mixed form of cell death with signs of necrosis, also called "secondary necrosis" [45, 65, 68, 91]. Therefore, it is not surprising that histochemical analyses clearly demonstrate the presence of necrotic as well as of apoptotic myocyte nuclei in ischemic myocardium with obvious ATP deficits [37] and in terminally failing overloaded myocardium [30], in which intramyocyte losses of mitochondria and contractile filaments may occur [23, 80]. The presence of myocytes with nuclear and extranuclear signs of necrosis does not yield a strong argument against a major role of the apoptotic program as a contributor to myocyte losses.

On the other hand, however, definitive proof for the causal relevance of the apoptotic program in heart diseases cannot be obtained only from histochemical, ultrastructural or biochemical characterizations of myocyte nuclei and nuclear DNA. The limitations of such analyses are summarized in Table 1.

■ Experimental inhibitions of apoptosis suggest functional relevance of the program in cardiac pathologies

Recently, experimental data on the effect of apoptosis inhibition on myocyte losses and infarct size in models of permanent or transient myocardial ischemia have been summarized [4]. The conclusion was reached that in ischemia-associated myocardial perturbations the cardiomyocytes mainly succumb to mixed forms of cell death with substantial activations of the apoptotic program, but with more or less involvement of necrotic cytolysis [4]. The consequence of this "mixture" of ischemia-associated forms of myocyte death is that the release of cytosolic myocyte elements into the blood (clearly a necrotic step) predicts the size of myocardial infarction, but that antiapoptotic interventions in experimental models of ischemia attenuate or retard cell losses. Meanwhile, further data on the protective effect of anti-apoptotic interventions in experimental models of ischemia-associated myocardial damage have been published (Table 2). These most recent data support the concept that elements of programmed death substantially contribute to ischemia-associated losses of cardiomyocytes. Variabilities in the "mixture" of necrotic and apoptotic elements in myocyte death do exist depending on the species, the model and the involvement of postischemic reperfusion. However, these experimental analyses clearly document the functional relevance of the apoptotic program for the consequences of myocardial ischemia, confirming the suggestions obtained from histochemical and biochemical analyses. In myocardial ischemia, apoptosis is more than an irrelevant epiphenomenon!

Concerning the effects of antiapoptotic interventions in overload-associated cardiac failure, very few experimental data are available. Insulin-like growth factor I (IGF-I) has been characterized as a potent antiapoptotic fac-

Table 2. Protective efficacy of anti-apoptotic interventions in myocardial ischemia-associated damage (recent experimental data)

Model	Anti-apoptotic intervention	Protective effect	Ref.
Cultured neonatal rat cardiomyocytes with simulated ischemia (hypoxia/reox.)	Adenovirus-mediated coexpression of hsp60 and hsp10	–20% LDH release; –27% TUNEL stained myocytes; attenuated mitochondrial loss of cytochrome c	[53]
Rat heterotopic heart transplantation model with ischemia (30')/reperfusion (45')	Transfection by double stranded p53 decoy DNA	–48% infarct size by nitro blue tetrazolium staining with reduced DNA laddering and Bax expression	[17]
Rabbit heart ischemia (30')/reperfusion (4 h) in vivo	Adenovirus-mediated overexpression of Bcl-2 +catalase, one week prior to ischemia	–78% apoptosis; –77% infarct size; postischemic fractional shortening improved from 36 to 75%	[93]
Isolated perfused working rat heart with ischemia (30')/reperfusion (30')	Perfusion with specific inhibitors of caspase 1 or caspase 3	Improved postischemic recovery of developed LV-pressure, contractility and cardiac work	[74]
Isolated perfused rat heart with ischemia (35')/reperfusion (120')	Perfusion with broad spectrum caspase inhibitor or caspase 9 inhibitor	Reduction in infarct size (relative to area at risk)	[60]
Ischemia/reperfusion in mice in vivo	Adenovirus-mediated expression of constitutively active Akt protein kinase	Reduction in ischemia-reperfusion induced myocyte apoptosis	[26]

tor in tumor cells, activating the Akt protein kinase survival pathway via the IGF receptor type I [6, 7, 27]. Cardiac overexpression of IGF-I in mice not only partially protects from myocyte death due to coronary ligation, but also attenuates dilatory remodelling in the nonischemic ventricular area remote from the infarction [51]. This protective effect for the nonischemic area cannot be explained by the IGF-I-induced reduction of infarct size, but is probably due to the reduction of load-induced apoptosis [51]. However, this cardiac IGF-I overexpression also results in cardiac enlargement with an augmented number of cardiomyocytes due to modifications of prenatal organogenesis [73]. Therefore, the enhanced resistance of this IGF-I transfected myocardium against overload-induced failure might have more complex reasons. In an experimental model of heart failure with ventricular dilation, induced by chronic ventricular tachypacing, growth hormone supplementation induced enhanced ventricular IGF-I expression, attenuated ventricular dilation and improved ventricular function [34]. In this experimental model of heart failure, cardiomyocyte apoptosis has been documented previously [39, 54]. Unfortunately, however, in the study on growth hormone supplementation, myocyte apoptosis was not evaluated [34].

Thus, the functional relevance of apoptotic cardiomyocyte losses, histochemically demonstrable in overloaded, nonischemic myocardium, is not yet definitely established by experimental studies with inhibitors of apoptosis. Probably, the pathologic role of apoptosis in overload-associated myocardial failure is due less to myocyte losses, but due more to functional myocyte impairment by preapoptotic alterations.

▦ Reversible cytosolic preapoptosis and postmitochondrial retardation of nuclear apoptosis in failing myocardium

Release of the diffusible respiratory chain protein cytochrome c from the intermembrane space of the mitochondria is an important step in the apoptotic program (Fig. 1) and is observed in cardiomyocytes upon myocardial ischemia [22, 53]. In explanted ventricles from patients with terminal heart failure, there is substantial cytochrome c release in myocytes from nonischemic, overloaded ventricular areas [64]. This release is demonstrated as extramitochondrial localization of cytochrome c by ultrastructural histochemistry and by Western blot analyses in tissue extracts. Furthermore, cytosolic consequences of this cytochrome c release are documented: the terminal effector caspase 3 is cleaved (which is an indirect indicator of activation of the caspase cascade) as well as a cytosolic substrate of these activated caspases, the protein kinase Cδ (PKCδ) [64].

The remarkable aspects of these findings are quantitative relations: while roughly 55% of the total myocardial cytochrome c was located extramitochondrially and >50% of cytosolic caspase 3 or PKCδ was cleaved, no cleavage of the nuclear caspase substrate PARP (see Fig. 2) could be detected by Western blot techniques [64]. PARP, however, is considered as an ideal "marker" of nuclear apoptotic processes. This means that in terminally failing human myocardium, in which some 0.2% of myocytes demonstrate histochemical signs of nuclear apoptosis [66, 76], and in which cleavage of nuclear PARP is still below the level of biochemical detection, there is strong activation of mitochondrial and cytosolic steps of the program! A comparable "delay" between cytosolic/mitochondrial preapoptosis and nuclear apoptosis has never been observed in any other tissue or cell type. This "dissociation" of the program triggered a search for cardiomyocyte-specific postmitochondrial regulators of apoptosis, which could mediate this remarkable retardation of the program in failing human hearts [72]. While several candidate proteins can be discussed as mediators of this retardation [72], the issue is still entirely unresolved.

Which potential consequences for cardiomyocyte function might result from the release of more than 50% of mitochondrial cytochrome c? Three possibilities have to be considered:

▩ reduced respiratory maximal capacity of the respiratory chain due to a substantial reduction in the mitochondrial content of the diffusible respiratory chain protein cytochrome c

▩ enhanced mitochondrial radical formation because of a partially defective respiratory chain in the presence of normal oxygenation

▩ altered regulatory signaling or contractile performance due to cleavage of cytosolic caspase substrates such as PKCδ [63], troponin C [31, 52] or others.

The most obvious functional impairment could be guessed to result from the diminished respiratory capacity of the mitochondria in the failing heart. Ironically, however, it is not clear to what extent mitochondria might contain an excess of diffusible cytochrome c relative to the capacity of the other elements of the respiratory chain. Therefore, the extent in the decline of respiratory capacity cannot be predicted for myocyte mitochondria with a more than 50% deficit of cytochrome c, although it appears unlikely that any mitochondrial excess content of cytochrome c should amount to such a degree that a 50% loss should be tolerable without impairments.

A respiratory chain with a relevant deficit of cytochrome c, however, should produce more reactive oxygen species as long as tissue oxygen pressure is not lowered [42, 43, 85]. This should contribute to further mitochondrial damage.

Finally, caspase-mediated cleavage of cytosolic substrates, triggered by cytochrome c-induced activation of initiator caspases, might exceed the rate of *de novo* synthesis of these substrates. The majority of cyotosolic substrates of activated caspases in cardiomyocytes remain to be identified. However, it is tempting to speculate that the deficit in contractile fibers and the cytoskeletal alterations, documented by ultrastructural analyses in terminal heart failure [80], are a consequence of the strong cytosolic activation of the proteolytic caspase cascade with enhanced degradation of caspase substrates such as troponin C [31, 52].

The detailed mechanisms of mitochondrial release of cytochrome c (and of other apoptogens) from the intermembrane space is under extensive research at pesent and several mechanisms appear to exist, depending on cell type and apoptotic stimulus. In mitochondria from several cell types, release can occur without irreversible rupture of mitochondrial membranes and destruction of mitochondrial structures [9, 10, 83]. Similarly, the mitochondria in the failing human heart with 50% extramitochondrial cytochrome c did not demonstrate obvious signs of structural abnormalities in electronmicroscopic micrographs [64]. In this context it is important to note that in rather terminally differentiated cells such as cortical neurons, apoptotic cytochrome c release is a reversible process, since mitochondrial reuptake of the released holoenzyme was documented [59].

Although mitochondrial reuptake of released cytochrome c within cardiomyocytes remains to be illustrated in detail, the basic reversibility of the process [59] together with the cardiospecific retardation in the transfer of the apoptotic process to the myocyte nuclei [72] suggests that the functionally important part of the apoptotic activation in overloaded, failing cardiomyocytes is the reversible, cytosolic preapoptosis. This process might turn out to be much more important than the irrevesible nucleolysis and DNA degradation. There is good reason to expect that the focus in myocardial apoptosis research will be shifted away from counting TUNEL-stained nuclei with speculations on tissue "melting rates". Instead, the focus will be turned towards the substantially and functionally important reversible processes in myocyte cytosol and mitochondria.

Since the definition of apoptosis requires typical DNA cleavage, these reversible processes cannot be called apoptotic, although elements of the program are activated. Therefore, the term "reversible preapoptosis" appears appropriate.

Provided that the stimulus for myocyte apoptosis is removed by therapy, the reuptake of cytochrome c into the mitochondria should terminate the activation of the caspase cascade. Subsequently, *de novo* protein synthesis could replace caspase-cleaved cytosolic substrates with full restoration of myocyte function. The critical question is whether the apoptogenic stimulus in a terminally failing heart can be really removed.

■ Hemodynamic unloading by ventricluar assist devices: A clinical experiment for reversibility of failure associated myocardial alterations

It is generally assumed that overload-induced phenotype changes in the failing myocardium result from altered gene expression in response to distension of the cardiomyocytes [41, 69]. Distension of cultured cardiomyocytes from neonatal or adult rodents has been successfully used as a cellular model to obtain insights into signaling pathways of distension-induced phenotype changes [75]. These models have also been used to demonstrate distension-induced apoptosis in cultured cardiomyocytes [47, 48]. While such cellular models are indispensable for the evaluation of cellular and molecular mechanisms of the process under study, the relevance of findings from these cellular models for the intact organ will always remain some matter of debate. This is especially true for the issue of apoptosis in cardiomyocytes, which occurs at a very high basal rate in cardiomyocytes in culture without any apoptotic stimulus.

Experimental models with induction and removal of enhanced cardiac load in vivo have not yet been used for the analysis of reversibility of pre-apoptotic activations in response to overload. However, the hemodynamic unloading obtained by the implantation of ventricular assist devices yields an excellent clinical opportunity to look for overload-associated phenotype plasticity in human myocardium. These devices are usually installed in patients with terminal heart failure, in which cardiac function cannot be stabilized otherwise [25, 36, 49]. In general, the intention is to bridge the time until availability of a nonfailing donor heart by the cardiac unloading and cardiac support supplied by the assist device, working in parallel with the failing ventricle [55, 82]. With the implantation of the device, an apical part from the terminally failing ventricle must be removed for installation of the inlet of the artificial pump, and this specimen of failing myocardium is available for phenotype analysis. Later, when a donor heart is available, and when some recovery of peripheral organs has occurred, the failing heart is explanted, yielding further specimens of the same ventricle for phenotype analysis after a period of hemodynamic unloading.

Table 3. Renormalization of heart failure-typical cardiac abnormalities under VAD-induced hemodynamic unloading

Renormalization of tissue or myocyte phenotype under VAD	Ref.
1) Leftward shift of diastolic LV pressure-volume curves in arrested hearts; Enddiastolic pressure volume relationship renormalized, with an optimum of structural recovery between 40 and 100 days of support;	[50] [57, 62]
2) Reduction of cardiomyocyte hypertrophy and myofiber thickness;	[21, 62, 92]
3) Normalization of enhanced ventricular ProANP expression, considered as a marker of cardiomyocyte overload hypertrophy;	[5]
4) Reduction in interstitial fibrosis and collagen III staining in four patients with successful weaning from VAD support;	[62]
5) Upregulation of depressed SERCA expression at the level of mRNA, protein or function in subgroups of VAD-supported patients;	[5, 24, 87]
6) Reduction of enhanced ET_A receptor mRNA expression;	[61]
7) Normalization of reduced mRNA expression of glucose transportes GLUT1 and GLUT4;	[18, 19]
8) Reduced protein expression of RGS2 (regulator of G protein signaling 2), the selective inhibitor of $G\alpha q$.	[87]

Such a comparison of specimens in pairs from the same heart has been used repeatedly for the analysis of phenotype plasticity of cardiomyocytes in failing human myocardium. Table 3 demonstrates typical features of failing human myocardium, which have been shown to be partially renormalized under the unloading obtained by assist devices. Furthermore, a substantial decline in ventricular DNA-"laddering" (i.e., apoptotic DNA cleavage into nucleosome-sized fragments) has been observed in failing hearts under the support by assist device, suggesting a substantial decline in the ongoing rate of nuclear apoptosis [5]. In Table 4, data from this analysis on device-induced changes in apoptosis regulation are listed together with other changes under the assist device, which might affect the susceptibility of failing cardiomyocytes to apoptosis.

These preliminary data, demonstrating the renormalized expression of anti-apoptotic inhibitors, the renormalization of mitochondrial function and structure components, and the disappearance in the local expression of TNFa and iNOS (i.s., inducible NO synthase) strongly suggest that an enhanced susceptiblity in the failing hearts prior to the installation of the assist device is reduced again under the support obtained by this device (Table 4). Therefore, the extent of cytosolic/mitochondrial preapoptosis in the terminally failing myocardium and its reversibility by unloading is presently under study in this important clinical model. We expect this study to demonstrate that cytosolic preapoptosis, the functionally and quantitatively important aspect of apoptosis in failing cardiomyocytes, is indeed reversible.

However, several caveats have to be kept in mind! First of all, and most importantly: the reversibility of cytosolic preapoptosis in failing cardiomyocytes is nothing but a working hypothesis, maybe a plausible and attractive one, but nevertheless still speculative!

Second, assuming that cytosolic preapoptosis is reversible upon cardiac unloading by assist devices, this would not yet prove the functional relevance of the process for the deterioration of cardiac function in the failing heart. To this end, experimental models of cardiac overload with inhibition of cytosolic preapoptosis would be desirable.

Furthermore, chronic hemodynamic support by assist devices is not only a renormalization of exaggerated loading conditions for the failing heart, but it has to be assumed that there is also some renormalization of the augmented neuroendocrine activity and, probably, some alteration in the degree of systemic inflammatory activation. Therefore, assist device-induced changes in the failing heart cannot be ascribed alone to the altered cardiac mechanics.

Finally, all data listed in Tables 3 and 4 have the character of anecdotical observations. These data are selected from small subgroups out of all those patients, in which the application of the devices was started. In these subsets of patients, the application of the assist device resulted in the successful stabilization, so that the device really had acted as a bridge to transplantation or even to functional recovery without the necessity of further

Table 4. Myocardial apoptosis and expression of regulators of apoptosis susceptibility under VAD support

VAD-induced alteration	Ref.	Relation to apoptosis regulation	Ref.
1) Reduction in LV "DNA ladder" score (parameter for nucleosome-sized DNA fragmentation)	[5]	Nuclear apoptosis is characterized by internucleosomal DNA cleavage	[15, 70]
2) Enhanced expression of bcl-x_L and mcl-1 (upregulation of bcl-x_L correlating with time on VAD support)	[5]	Bcl-x_L and Mcl-1 are antiapoptotic proteins of the Bcl-2 family, which inhibit mitochondrial inner membrane depolarization and cytochrome c release	[1, 71]
3) Enhanced mRNA expression of Fas antagonist FasExo6Del (upregulation correlating with time on VAD support)	[5]	Soluble Fas isoforms (e.g., Fas-Exo6Del) attenuate Fas-induced apoptosis in cell models by binding and inactivating Fas-ligand	[13]
4) Reduction of enhanced cardiac TNFα expression	[19, 90]	TNFα can induce cell death and/or inhibit myocyte contractile performance via death-domain-containing TNF type I receptors	[89]
5) Reduction of enhanced cardiac iNOS expression	[19]	Ca^{++}-induced activation of mitochondrial NOS mediates cytochrome c release (mtNOS probably related with iNOS)	[29]
6) Improved mitochondrial function (respiratory control index) and structure (cardiolipin isoform shift)	[33, 46]	Disturbances in respiratory chain function tend to promote mitochondrial radical formation, uncoupling and release of apoptogenic factors	[84, 86]

assist or subsequent transplantation [62]. Thus, these data do not show that myocardial recovery is a general response of failing myocardium under assist devices! However, these data on the upregulation of several endogenous inhibitors of apoptotic cytochrome c release under VAD support suggest that the extent of reversibility of cytosolic apoptosis can by quantitated in this model. This quantification, on the other hand, might turn out to be a valuable indicator of functional recovery of failing myocardium under assist device mediated support.

■ **Acknowledgment.** Our own studies mentioned in this report were supported by grants of the German Bundesministerium für Bildung und Forschung (BMBF, 01ZZ9512.TV3 & TV7).

■ References

1. Adams JM, Cory S (1998) The Bcl-2 protein family: arbiters of cell survival. Science 281:1322–1325
2. Anversa P, Kajstura J (1998) Myocyte cell death in the diseased heart. Circ Res 82:1231–1233
3. Anversa P, Kajstura J, Reiss K, Quaini F, Baldini A, Olivetti G, Sonnenblick EH (1995) Ischemic cardiomyopathy: myocyte cell loss, myocyte cellular hypertrophy, and myocyte cellular hyperplasia. Ann NY Acad Sci 752:47–64
4. Bartling B, Holtz J, Darmer D (1998) Contribution of myocyte apoptosis to myocardial infarction? Basic Res Cardiol 93:71–84
5. Bartling B, Milting H, Schumann H, Darmer D, Arusoglu L, Koerner MM, El-Banayosy A, Koerfer R, Holtz J, Zerkowski HR (1999) Myocardial gene expression of regulators of myocyte apoptosis and myocyte calcium homeostasis during hemodynamic unloading by ventricular assist devices in patients with end-stage heart failure. Circulation 100 (Suppl II):II216–II223
6. Baserga R, Hongo A, Rubini M, Prisco M, Valentinis B (1997) The IGF-I receptor in cell growth, transformation and apoptosis. Biochim Biophys Acta 1332:F105–F126
7. Baserga R, Resnicoff M, Dews M (1997) The IGF-I receptor and cancer. Endocrine 7:99–102
8. Bing OHL (1994) Hypothesis: apoptosis may be a mechanism for the transition to heart failure with chronic pressure overload. J Mol Cell Cardiol 26:943–948
9. Bossy-Wetzel E, Green DR (1999) Caspases induce cytochrome c release from mitochondria by activating cytosolic factors. J Biol Chem 274:17484–17490
10. Bossy-Wetzel E, Newmeyer DD, Green DR (1998) Mitochondrial cytochrome c release in apoptosis occurs upstream of DEVD-specific caspase activation and independently of mitochondrial transmembrane depolarization. Embo J 17:37–49
11. Brömme HJ, Holtz J (1996) Apoptosis in the heart: when and why? Molecular and Cellular Biochemistry 163/164:261–275
12. Budihardjo I, Oliver H, Lutter M, Luo X, Wang X (1999) Biochemical pathways of caspase activation during apoptosis. Ann Rev Cell Dev Biol 15:269–290
13. Cascino I, Papoff G, De Maria R, Testi R, Ruberti G (1996) Fas/Apo-1 (CD95) receptor lacking the intracytoplasmic signaling domain protects tumor cells from Fas-mediated apoptosis. J Immunol 156:13–17

14. Cheng W, Li B, Kajstura J, Li P, Wolin MS, Sonnenblick EH, Hintze TH, Olivetti G, Anversa P (1995) Stretch induced programmed myocyte cell death. J Clin Invest 96:2247–2259

15. Collins RJ, Harmon BV, Gove GC, Kerr JFR (1992) Internucleosomal DNA cleavage should not be the sole criterion for identifying apoptosis. Int J Radiat Biol 61:451–453

16. Cook SA, Poole-Wilson PA (1999) Cardiac myocyte apoptosis. Eur Heart J 28:1619–1629

17. Dell'Acqua G, Mann MJ, Zhang LN, Ehsan A, Dzau VJ (1999) Ex vivo gene therapy with p53 transcription factor decoy attenuates apoptosis and myocardial damage in a rat model of ischemia/reperfusion (abstr). Circulation 100 (Suppl I):I-481

18. Depre C, Shipley GL, Davies PJA, Frazier OH, Taegtmeyer H (1998) Glucose transporter isoform expression in the failing human heart (abstr). Circulation 98 (Suppl I):I-827

19. Depre C, Shipley GL, Frazier OH, Davies PJ, Taegtmeyer H (1999) Reprogramming of dysfunctional gene expression after mechanical unloading in failing human heart (abstr). Circulation 100 (Suppl I):I-802

20. Didenko VV, Hornby PJ (1996) Presence of double-stranded breaks with single-base 3' overhangs in cells undergoing apoptosis but not necrosis. J Cell Biol 135:1369–1376

21. Dipla K, Mattiello JA, Jeevanandam V, Houser SR, Mardulies KB (1998) Myocyte recovery after mechanical circulatory support in humans with endstage heart failure. Circulation 97:2316–23322

22. Fan THM, Xu J, Pain TS, Krenz M, Cohen MV, Downey JM (1999) Diazoxide inhibits mitochondrial cytochrome c release in ischemic rabbit myocardium (abstr). Circulation 100 (Suppl I):I-630

23. Figulla HR, Rahlf G, Nieger M, Luig H, Kreuzer H (1985) Spontaneous hemodynamic improvement or stabilization and associated biopsy findings in patients with congestive cardiomyopathy. Circulation 71:1095–1104

24. Frazier H, Benedict CR, Radovancevic B, Bick RJ, Capek P, Springer WE, Marcis MP, Delgado R, Buja M (1998) Improved left ventricular function after chronic left ventricular unloading. Ann Thorac Surg 62:675–682

25. Frazier OH, Rose EA, McCarthy P (1995) Improved mortality and rehabilitation of transplant candidates treated with a long term implantable left-ventricular assist system. Ann Thorac Cardiovasc Surg 222:327–338

26. Fujio K, Mano T, Takahashi T, Walsh K (1998) Akt mediates the cell survival effects of vascular endothelial growth factor (abstr). Circulation 98 (Suppl-I):I-463

27. Fujio Y, Kitsis RN, Walsh K (1999) Akt mediates IGF-1 cytoprotection of cardiomyocytes in vitro and protects against ischemi-reperfusion injury in mouse heart (abstr). Circulation 100 (Suppl I):I-9

28. Gavrieli Y, Shermann Y, Ben-Sasson SA (1992) Identification of programmed cell death in situ via specific labeling of nuclear DNA fragmentation. J Cell Biol. 119:493–501

29. Ghafourifar P, Schenk U, Klein SD, Richter C (1999) Mitochondrial nitric-oxide synthase stimulation causes cytochrome c release from isolated mitochondria: evidence for intramitochondrial peroxynitrite formation. J Biol Chem 274:31185–31188

30. Guerra S, Leri A, Wang X, Finato N, Di Loreto C, Beltrami CA, Kajstura J, Anversa P (1999) Myocyte death in the failing human heart is gender dependent. Circ Res 85:856–866

31 Haider N, Kharbanda S, Chandrasekar Y, Srinivasula SM, Fitzpatrick JM, Anand I, Alnemri ES, Narula J (1999) Caspase-3 mediated cleavage of troponin-C at evolutionarily conserved calcium binding site: relevance of apoptosis in heart failure (abstr). Circulation 100 (Suppl):I-283

32. Haunstetter A, Izumo S (1998) Apoptosis: basic mechanisms and implications for cardiovascular disease. Circ Res 82:1111–1129

33. Heerdt PM, Choudhri AF, Scvhlame M (1999) Left ventricular assist devices promote mitochondrial remodeling in ischemic but not idiopathic dilated cardiomyopathy. Circulation 100 (Suppl I):I–167 (abstr.)

34. Houck WV, Pan LC, Kribbs SB, Clair MJ, McDaniel GM, Krombach S, Merritt WM, Pirie C, Iannini JP, Mukherjee R, Spinale FG (1999) Effects of growth hormone supplementation on left ventricular morphology and myocyte function with the development of congestive heart failure. Circulation 1000:2003–2009

35. James TN (1994) Normal and abnormal consequences of apoptosis in the human heart from postnatal morphogenesis to paroxysmal arrhythmias. Circulation 90:556–573

36. Jaski BE, Kim J, Maly RS, Branch KR, Adamson R, Favrot LK, Smith SC, Dembitsky WP (1997) Effects of exercise during long-term support with a left ventricular assist device: results of the experience with left ventricular assist device with exercise (EVADE) pilot trial. Circulation 95:2401–2406

37. Kajstura J, Cheng W, Reiss K, Clark WA, Sonnenblick EH, Krajeski S, Reed JC, Olivetti G, Anversa P (1995) Apoptotic and necrotic myocyte cell death are independent contributing variables of infarct size in rats. Lab Invest 74:86–107

38. Kajstura J, Leri A, Finato N, Di Loreto C, Beltrami CA, Anversa P (1998) Myocyte proliferation in end-stage cardiac failure in humans. Proc Natl Acad Sci 95:8801–8805

39. Kajstura J, Zhang X, Liu Y, Szoke E, Cheng W, Olivetti G, Hintze TH, Anversa P (1995) The cellular basis of pacing-induced dilated cardiomyopathy: myocyte cell loss and myocyte cellular reactive hypertrophy. Circulation 92:2306–2317

40. Kanoh M, Takemura G, Misao J, Hayakawa Y, Aoyama T, Nishigaki K, Noda T, Fujiwara T, Fukuda F, Minatoguchi S, Fujiwara H (1999) Significance of myocytes with positive DNA in situ nick end-labeling (TUNEL) in hearts with dilated cardiomyopathy: not apoptosis but DNA repair. Circulation 99:2757–2764

41. Katz AM (1994) The cardiomyopathy of overload: an unnatural growth response in the hypertrophied heart. Ann Intern Med 121:363–371

42. Korshunov SS, Krasnikov BF, Pereverzev MO, Skulachev VP (1999) The antioxidant functions of cytochrome c. FEBS Lett 462:192–198

43. Korshunov SS, Skulachev VP, Starkov AA (1997) High protonic potential actuates a mechanism of production of reactive oxygen species in mitochondria. FEBS Lett 416:15–18

44. Kroemer G (1997) Mitochondrial implication in apoptosis: towards an endosymbiont hypothesis of apoptosis evolution. Cell Death Diff 4:443–456

45. Kroemer G, Dallaporta B, Resche-Rigon M (1998) The mitochondrial death/life regulator in apoptosis and necrosis. Ann Rev Physiol 60:619–642

46. Lee SH, Doliba N, Osbakken M, Oz M, Mancini D (1998) Improvement of myocardial mitochondrial function after hemodynamic support with left ventricular assist devices in patients with heart failure. J Thorac Cardiovasc Surg 116:344–349

47. Leri A, Claudio PP, Li Q, Wang X, Reiss K, Wang S, Malhotra A, Kajstura J, Anversa P (1998) Stretch-mediated release of angiotensin II induces myocyte apoptosis by activating p53 that enhances the local renin-angiotensin system and decreases the bcl-2-to-bax ratio in the cell. J Clin Invest 101:1326–1342

48. Leri A, Liu Y, Claudio PP, Kajstura J, Wang X, Wang S, Kang P, Malhotra A, Anversa P (1999) Insulin-like growth factor-1 induces Mdm2 and downregulates p53, attenuating the myocyte renin-angiotensin system and stretch-mediated apoptosis. Am J Pathol 154:567–580

49. Levin HR, Chen JM, Oz MC (1994) Potential of left ventricular assist devices as outpatient therapy while awaiting transplantation. Ann Thorac Surg 58:1515–1520

50. Levin HR, Oz MC, Chen JM, Packer M, Rose EA, Burkhoff D (1995) Reversal of chronic ventricular dilation in patients with endstage cardiomyopathy by prolonged mechanical unloading. Circulation 91:2717–2720

51. Li Q, Li B, Wang X, Levi A, Jana KP, Liu X, Kajstura J, Baserga R, Anversa P (1997) Overexpression of insulin growth factor-1 in mice protects from myocyte death after infarction, attenuating ventricular dilation, wall stress and cardiac hypertrophy. J Clin Invest 100:1991–1999

52. Liao R, Gwathmey JK, Wang CK (1999) A possible mechanism for decreased myocardial contractility in idiopathic dilated cardiomyopathy: significance of spatial relationship between Helix A and Ca2+-binding loop II in human cardiac troponin C (abstr). Circulation 100 (suppl):II-60

53. Lin KM, Mestril R, Dillamnn WH (1999) Mitochondrial chaperonins protect cardiac myocytes against apoptotic cell death induced by ischemia-reoxygenation (abstr). Circulation 100 (Suppl I):I-838

54. Liu Y, Cigola E, Cheng W, Kajastura J, Olivetti G, Hintze TH, Anversa P (1995) Myocyte nuclear mitotic division and programmed myocyte cell death characterize the cardiac myopathy induced by rapid ventricular pacing in dogs. Lab Invest 73:771–787

55. Loebe M, Müller J, Hetzer R (1999) Ventricular assistance for recovery of cardiac failure. Curr Opin Cardiol 14:234–248

56. MacLellan WR, Schneider MD (1997) Death by design: programmed cell death in cardiovascular biology and disease. Circ Res 81:137–144

57. Madigan JD, Choudhri AF, Morales DLS, Burkhoff D, Oz MC (1999) The time course of reverse structural remodeling of the left ventricule during LVAD support. Circulation 100 (Suppl I):I-802 (abstr.)

58. Majno G, Joris I (1995) Apoptosis, oncosis, and necrosis. Am J Pathol 146:3–15

59. Martinou I, Desagher S, Eskes R, Antonsson B, Andre E, Fakan S, Martinou JC (1999) The release of cytochrome c from mitochondria during apoptosis of NGF-deprived sympathetic neurons is a reversible event. J Cell Biol 144:883–889

60. Mocanu MM, Baxter GF, Yellon DM (1999) Caspase inhibition at reperfusion protects the isolated rat heart (abstr). Circulation 100 (Suppl I):I-10

61. Morawietz H, Bartling B, Milting H, Schumann H, Darmer D, Holtz J, El-Banayosy A, Koerner MM, Koerfer R, Zerkowski HR (1999) Renormalization of endothelin receptor A expression under support by ventricular assist devices in patients with terminal heart failure (abstr). Circulation 100 (Suppl I):I-167

62. Müller J, Wallukat G, Weng YG, Dandel M, Spiegelsberger S, Semrau S, Brandes K, Theodoridis V, Loebe M, Meyer R, Hetzer R (1997) Weaning from mechanical cardiac support in patients with idiopathic dilated cardiomyopathy. Circulation 96:542–549

63. Narula J, Haider N, Virmani R, DiSalvo T, Kolodgie FD, Hajjar RJ, Schmidt U, Semigran MJ, Dec W, Khaw BA (1996) Apoptosis in myocytes in end-stage heart failure. N Engl J Med 335:1182–1189

64. Narula J, Pandey P, Arbustini E, Haider N, Narula N, Kolodgie FD, Dal Bello B, Semigran MJ, Bielsa-Madeu A, Dec GW, Israels S, Ballester M, Virmani R, Saxena S, Kharbanda S (1999) Apoptosis in heart failure: release of cytochrome c from mitochondria and activation of caspase-3 in human cardiomyopathy. Proc Natl Acad Sci 96:8144–8149

65. Nicotera P, Leist P (1997) Energy supply and the shape of death in neurons and lymphoid cells. Cell Death Diff 4:435–442

66 Olivetti G, Abbi R, Quaini F, Kajstura J, Cheng W, Nitahara JA, Quaini E, DiLoreto C, Beltrami CA, Krajewski S, Reed JC, Anversa P (1997) Apoptosis in the failing human heart. N Engl J Med 336:1131–1141

67. O'Rourke B (1999) Apoptosis: rekindling the mitochondrial fire. Circ Res 85:880–883
68. Orrenius S, Burgess DH, Hampton MB, Zhivotovsky B (1997) Mitochondria as the focus of apoptosis research. Cell Death Diff 4:427–428
69. Parker TG, Schneider MD (1991) Growth factors, proto-oncogenes, and plasticity of the cardiac phenotype. Ann Rev Physiol 53:179–200
70. Raff M (1998) Cell suicide for beginners. Nature 396:119–122
71. Reed JC (1997) Double identity for proteins of the Bcl-2 family. Nature 387:773–776
72. Reed JC, Paternostro G (1999) Postmitochondrial regulation of apoptosis during heart failure. Proc Natl Acad Sci 96:7614–7616
73. Reiss K, Kajstura J, Capasso JM, Marino TA, Anversa P (1993) Impairment of myocyte contractility following coronary artery narrowing is associated with activation of the myocyte IGF autocrine system, enhanced expression of late growth related genes, DNA-synthesis and myocyte nuclear mitotic division in rats. Exp Cell Res 207:348–360
74. Ruetten H, Dimmeler S (1999) Caspase inhibitors improve post–ischemic functional recovery in isolated rat working hearts (abstr). Circulation 100 (Suppl I):I–10
75. Sadoshima J, Izumo S (1997) The cellular and molecular response of cardiac myocytes to mechanical stress. Ann Rev Physiol 59:551–571
76. Saraste A, Pulkki K, Kallajoki M, Heikkilä P, Laine P, Mattila S, Nieminen MS, Parvinen M, Voipio-Pulkki LM (1999) Cardiomyocyte apoptosis and progression of heart failure to transplantation. Eur J Clin Invest 29:380–386
77. Saraste A, Pulkki K, Kallajoki M, Henriksen K, Parvinen M, Voipio-Pulkki LM (1997) Apoptosis in human acute myocardial infarction. Circulation 95:320–323
78. Scaffidi C, Fulda S, Srinivasan A, Friesen C, Li F, Tomaselli KJ, Debatin KM, Krammer PH, Peter ME (1998) Two CD95 (APO-1/Fas) signaling pathways. EMBO J 17:1675–1687
79. Schaper J, Elsässer A, Kostin S (1999) The role of cell death in heart failure. Circ Res 85:867–869
80. Schaper J, Froede R, Hein S, Buck A, Hashizume H, Speiser B, Briedl A, Bleese N (1991) Impairment of the myocardial ultrastructure and changes of the cytoskeleton in dilated cardiomyopathy. Circulation 83:504–514
81. Schaper J, Lorenz–Meyer S, Suzuki K (1999) The role of apoptosis in dilated cardiomyopathy. Herz 24:219–224
82. Scheld HH (1996) Mechanical support: benefits and risks. Thorac cardiovasc surgeon 45:1–5
83. Shimizu S, Narita M, Tsujimoto Y (1999) Bcl-2 family proteins regulate the release of apoptogenic cytochrome c by the mitochondrial channel VDAC. Nature 399:483–487
84. Skulachev PV (1998) Uncoupling. New approaches to an old problem of bioenergetics. Biochim Biophys Acta 1363:205–278
85. Skulachev VP (1996) Role of uncoupled and non-coupled oxidations in maintenance of safely low levels of oxygen and its one-electron reductants. Quart Rev Biophys 29:169–202
86. Skulachev VP (1997) Membrane-linked system preventing superoxide formation. Biosci Reports 17:347–366
87. Takeishi Y, Jalili T, Kirkpatrick DL, Wagner LE, Abraham WT, Walsh RA (1999) Differential alterations in Ca^{2+} cycling and Gαq signaling proteins after left ventricular assist device support in failing human hearts. Circulation 100 (Suppl I):I–419 (abstr.)
88. Thornberry NA, Lazebnik Y (1998) Caspases: enemies within. Science 281:1313–1316

89. Torre-Amione G, Bozkurt B, Deswal A, Mann DL (1999) An overview of tumor necrosis factor a and the failing human heart. Curr Opin Cardiol 14:206–210
90. Torre–Amione G, Stetson SJ, Youker KA, Durand JB, Radovancevic B, Delgado RM, Frazier OH, Entman ML, Noon GP (1999) Decreased expression of tumor necrosis factor-alpha in failing human myocardium after mechanical circulatory support: a potential mechanism for cardiac recovery. Circulation 100:1189–1193
91. Tsujimoto Y (1997) Apoptosis and necrosis: intracellular ATP levels as a determinant for cell death modes. Cell Death Diff 4:429–434
92. Zafeiridis A, Jeevanandam V, Houser SR, Margulies KB (1998) Regression of cellular hypertrophy after left ventricular assist device support. Circulation 98:656–662
93. Zhu HL, Taylor MD, Vijayasarathy C, Gardner TJ, Sweeney HL (1999) Overexpression of Bcl-2 and catalase by adenoviral genetransfer ameliorates myocardial reperfusion injury (abstr). Circulation 100 (suppl I):I-9–I-10

Author's address:

Prof. Dr. Jürgen Holtz
Institute of Pathophysiology
Martin-Luther University Halle-Wittenberg
Magdeburger-Str. 18
06097 Halle-Saale, Germany
E-mail: juergen.holtz@medizin.uni-halle.de